# STANDING PILATES

## Strengthen and Tone Your Body Wherever You Are

### JOAN BREIBART

**WILEY**

John Wiley & Sons, Inc.

D1119487

All photographs © Sarah Silver
Illustration on p. 25 © James Sheehan

Published by John Wiley & Sons, Inc., Hoboken, New Jersey
Published simultaneously in Canada

Standing Pilates® is a registered trademark owned by PhysicalMind, Inc.

Design and production by Navta Associates, Inc.

For general information about our other products and services, please contact our Customer Care Department within the United States at (800) 762-2974, outside the United States at (317) 572-3993 or fax (317) 572-4002.

Wiley also publishes its books in a variety of electronic formats. Some content that appears in print may not be available in electronic books. For more information about Wiley products, visit our web site at www.wiley.com.

*Library of Congress Cataloging-in-Publication Data:*
Breibart, Joan.
    Standing pilates : strengthen and tone your body wherever you are / Joan Breibart.
        p. cm.
    Includes bibliographical references and index.
    ISBN 0-471-56655-1 (paper: alk. paper)
1.   Pilates method. 2. Physical fitness. 3. Exercise. I. Title.
    RA781.B725 2004
    613.7'1—dc22                                                    2004005668

Printed in the United States of America

10  9  8  7  6  5  4  3  2

For Doug, Peter, and Roger

# Contents

Acknowledgments                                               ix

1    My Personal Pilates Story                                 1

2    What Is Pilates?                                          3

3    Smart Body Information                                    7

4    The Classical Mat                                        29

5    Being Vertical                                           43

6    The Standing Exercises                                   49

7    After Standing Pilates                                  141

Afterword                                                    145

Appendix A    Pilates and the PhysicalMind
              Institute                                      147

Appendix B    Osteoporosis and How Pilates
              Can Help                                       149

Appendix C    Testimonials on Standing Pilates              157

Appendix D    Certifying Pilates Studios                     161

Appendix E    Standing Pilates Instructors                   167

Appendix F    Certified Pilates Instructors                  195

Glossary                                                     215

Index                                                        219

# Acknowledgments

The author would like to thank the following individuals for their special contributions:

- Jack Scovil, my supportive and visionary literary agent, who saw the value of Standing Pilates

- Tom Miller, my editor, for his sound advice and guidance

- Sarah Silver, who photographed expertly the many subtleties of Standing Pilates exercises

- Marika Molnar, P.T., whose knowledge and anatomical expertise as the Institute Clinical Adviser gave me the understanding to evolve the Pilates Method

- Sophia Cannonier, Melanie Johnson, and Barbara Sampson, the lovely models who worked so well in front of the camera

- Cathy Hannan, general manager of the PhysicalMind Institute, and the Institute staff for their skills, support, and endurance during the development of this book

- Shannon Murphy, for her excellent comparison of the benefits of exercising vertically and horizontally

- Alasdair MacCrae, whose technical computer skills produced the exercise drawings for the professional course

- James Sheehan, for his drawing that describes our internal "domes"

- Mozhan Navabi, for editorial assistance in organizing the manuscript

- Eve Gentry, who shared what Joseph Pilates taught her

- Pat Grant, for her inspiring example of character

- My sons, Roger and Peter Bittenbender, for their daily help and advice

A very special thanks to Lesley Powell, whose movement abilities lent so much to the development of these exercises. Lesley owns Movements Afoot, the PhysicalMind Institute's certifying center in New York City. A fitness trainer since 1986, she is certified in Pilates and as a movement analyst from the Laban/Barteneiff Institute. Lesley holds a B.F.A. from Temple University, and has been on the faculty of Drew University since 1991, teaching classes in dance history, modern dance, and choreography.

My thanks also to our Certifying Teachers and the membership of the PhysicalMind Institute for their suggestions, encouragement, and devotion to the Pilates Method.

Joan Breibart, whose picture first appears on page 52, has practiced Pilates for four decades. In 1991 she founded the PhysicalMind Institute (formerly the Institute for the Pilates Method), which started the Pilates trend. After graduation from Barnard College, she spent a decade in publishing. She has developed, edited, and coauthored numerous books, including *Anatomy of Pilates* (PMI 2001). Subsequent careers were in consumer products marketing and services. DietDirectives, Pilates for the Palate (www.dietdirectives.com) is her current project.

Melanie Johnson, whose picture first appears on page 27 (top), owns Powerflow Pilates Studios, the PhysicalMind Institute's certifying center in New Haven, Connecticut. In addition to Pilates, she holds certifications from ACE, AAFA, AAAI/ISMA, Reiki II, and NIA. Melanie has studied dance and yoga for over twenty years. She is now training for Gyrotonic certification. She has been voted "Best Personal Trainer" in New Haven for the past four years.

Barbara Sampson, whose picture first appears on page 12, owned All About Movement, the PhysicalMind Institute's certifying center in Wellesley, Massachusetts. Barbara, a former competitive athlete, began Pilates training with Romana Kryzanova before becoming a certified trainer and later a teacher trainer for the institute. Barbara is also ACE and AAFA certified. She is the resident teacher trainer/examination director for the Institute.

Sophia Cannonier, whose picture first appears on page 8, owns the Health Corp, the PhysicalMind Institute's certifying center in Bermuda. Sophia is certified in Pilates, massage therapy, and Feldenkrais. A former Miss Bermuda, she performed with the Dance Theatre of Harlem until 1995. After an ankle injury halted her career, she began to study Pilates with Romana Kryzanova. She became an Institute teacher in 1999.

# 1

# My Personal
# Pilates Story

Today there are thousands of certified Pilates instructors in private studios, health clubs, physical therapy offices, hospitals, YMCAs, universities, dance studios, and spas—everywhere that people gather to gain better bodies. But when I began in the mid-sixties, there were only three Pilates studios in the world, all within a few blocks of one another in Manhattan. They were practically identical: the exercises, the equipment, the technique, and even the fees.

Despite its limited availability, Pilates had good press. There were major articles about Joseph Pilates in national magazines and New York newspapers. Joe's opinions in such quotes such as "Physical fitness is the first requisite for happiness," and "There is no hope for world peace if the members of the United Nations cannot do my first five mat exercises," were controversial, which attracted me. I decided to try Pilates, even though "working out" wasn't even a term back then. During the subsequent decades, I sampled the poplar fitness trends: running, Jazzercise, Nautilus, and even killer aerobics classes. Although I knew nothing about functional anatomy or correct biomechanics (and neither did the instructors), I never felt that the popular go-for-the-burn exercise mantra made sense.

I was still a Pilates fan when, in 1988, my family moved to Santa Fe, New Mexico. I had heard that there were some Pilates studios outside of New York, in California and London, but it was still such a secret. Pilates clients liked it that way, too. But at that time, leaving New York meant that I would have to leave Pilates.

Three years later, I was enjoying Santa Fe, but my body, particularly my neck and shoulders, definitely missed Pilates. A chiropractor told me that my neck was too "locked up" to release, but recommended a woman who did body miracles and had this funny exercise equipment. I called her immediately.

Her name was Eve Gentry and she had taught Pilates for Joe in his original studio since the mid-forties. After Joe's death in 1967, she had moved to Santa Fe and opened a Pilates practice with equipment that Clara, Joe's wife, had built especially for her. When I walked to her studio the next day, I had to go only three blocks. I had lived in Santa Fe for three years and she had been in my backyard!

Soon I was feeling good again and I began to think about how Pilates was so special and why no one knew about it. Between February and April 1991, I toyed with the idea of starting a professional organization to train instructors in the Pilates method. But I was on the fence until mid-April.

As I was reading the Sunday *New York Times*, an article by Penelope Green about exercise got my attention. It suggested that we had all tired of trying to be Jane Fonda and Arnold Schwarzenegger and maybe we should go back to the real stuff, Pilates. I took that as a sign that I should go ahead: April 14, 1991, was my fiftieth birthday.

The next day Eve Gentry and her associate, Michele Larsson, and I started the Institute for the Pilates Method. In that year we would publish the *Pilates Forum* and the first Pilates Reformer encyclopedia; create the Pilates video, *Working Out the Pilates Way*; and teach the first Pilates Certification Conference.

In 2001, I returned to New York. I replaced a car with my feet for transportation. I found my legs again. This was a big shift in awareness, which was the impetus to evolve Pilates.

# 2

# What Is Pilates?

That simple question is typically answered by this description: a system of exercises to strengthen and stretch the body and improve tone and posture. But, since this can be said of many exercise programs, why is Pilates so special?

Pilates has always been hard to define because it appears to be so effortless. Until very recently, the lack of an explanation was not an issue because nobody was asking. Americans were sold on aerobics, "going for the burn," and "no pain/no gain." When we started the Institute for the Pilates Method in 1991, we didn't know how to explain why Pilates worked. There were no research studies and despite its longevity, its reach had been minimal.

In the early 1990s while we were trying to capture the essence of Pilates in words, something happened that made this unnecessary. Stories started to appear that revealed the names of celebrities and dancers who were secret Pilates fans. Whether it was the famous names or the secrecy or both, the Pilates Method became an overnight success after seventy-five years. Joe Pilates had predicted that his method was fifty years ahead of its time and he was right.

Today Pilates terminology has been adopted by the very fitness world that had ignored and even ridiculed it for years. Now we hear that you need to crunch from the core. Aerobic routines are said to be total body exercise. And everything is body, mind, spirit.

Joe Pilates had many insights about the marvels of the human body, but my favorite had to do with watching animals. He explained, "Not even the laziest cat is out of shape. They stretch and tense their bodies, change positions often, and then go back to rest but stay in tune." Animals have a grace and a naturalness that is more than just muscle strength or speed. Joe noted the efficiency with which animals, big and small, use their bodies. He saw that when animals move, they use their entire bodies. These observations were the basis of *Contrology*, now known as Pilates, his body conditioning method. Its goal is a balanced body.

Pilates trains for natural, correct, and efficient movement. It requires us to pay attention. This is a starting point. Just awareness. Then we learn specific biomechanics (the study of forces on the skeleton and how they affect joint mobility and stability). Joints and muscles work together to create movement. Better bodies result from better-quality movement. Yes, you can get a better body by thinking correct thoughts. Form follows function. Sitting, eating, or watching TV is movement. If you are awake, you are moving.

Humans may look different, but anatomically we are the same in terms of muscles, bones, and ligaments. Yet some bodies look better and function better than others. We call these *smart bodies* because their brains deliver better movement information. At a very high level, we see that the physical abilities of Tiger Woods and Mikhail Baryshnikov are more than just good training. But do we recognize that other people who get results from exercises that don't work for us are beneficiaries of smart bodies, too?

Smart bodies can make dumb exercise functional and thus get results. Smart bodies can get a visual cue and translate it into correct movement. This is how Pilates used to be taught. Visualize that your spine is the shape of a ball and keep doing the exercise until your practice makes it perfect. It worked, too, for all those dancers and other great movers with smart bodies.

Smart bodies move as we were designed to function. For most people, this has to be learned or relearned because as adults we don't have this awareness. The real challenge is to develop a smart body, which translates into a better body and becomes a better-looking body. And you don't have to do hard workouts, either. You just need to pay attention to the right information, and gradually it will happen. How do I know? Because I did it in the past five years—proof that it is never too late to change. Surprised? Yes, I had decades of the old-style Pilates, and if I worked at it, I looked and felt better. But since

I didn't really know what was correct, my brain couldn't help me progress when I was not in the studio, which was 95 percent of the time.

This is an exercise book written by someone who is not a trainer, a coach, an athlete, or a dancer. Someone who, like most readers of exercise books, spends her days in front of a computer or sitting in a meeting—not in a gym, in a dance studio, or on a tennis court. The only difference between me and you is that I used my brain to change my body. Now I am going to tell you how to do it, and you should. It's your body, and if you don't pay attention to it, who will?

# 3

# Smart Body Information

Paying attention to your body begins with information learned in the Fundamentals and the Foundations. They are your passport to body-change. How were they discovered? Did Joseph Pilates use them? Why are they the basis of evolved Pilates?

## Eve Gentry: Early Pilates Teacher

When Eve Gentry moved to Santa Fe, she wanted to continue teaching the Pilates that she had learned. But the clients she saw were not able to do these complex movements. Some had injuries, so she began to work with them as Joe had with her when she injured her knee dancing with the Hanya Holm Company. And he helped her regain full motion of her arms after she had a radical mastectomy in the 1950s.

Eve had had other body training besides Pilates. She was a cofounder with Irmagard Bartenieff of the Dance Notation Bureau based on the work of Rudolph Laban, who pioneered a movement system and dance notation. Bartenieff, a physical and dance therapist who worked with Laban, focused on the "connections" inside the anatomy, not the obvious musculature. Eve then studied Feldenkrais, which deals with the neuromuscular pathways of the body.

Combining all of her body knowledge, Eve began to take apart the Pilates exercises to see what needed to happen for a nondancer to do complex movements. She experimented with doing the exercises more slowly than how she had learned them. Her analysis and experimentation became the basis of the Fundamentals, a sequence of minimovements to train body awareness.

## The Fundamentals

I have organized the Fundamentals by body segment. The Fundamentals are done in sequence, lying down with the knees bent and the pelvis in the neutral position. The torso has three Fundamentals: Neutral Spine, Breathing, and Pelvic Bowl. Then we move to the legs: Knee Fold, Knee Stir, Leg Slide, Knee Sway, and Bridging. Next is the Head Float. Finally, we have the arms: Rib Cage Arms and Arm Circles. Then we flip over to the front side of the body for Flight, Hip Extension, and Cat.

### Torso Fundamentals

Torso Fundamentals teach you what ideal posture feels like and how to isolate the top and bottom parts of your spine.

FUNDAMENTAL ONE: Neutral Spine

1. Lie on your back with your feet flat on the floor and your knees bent.

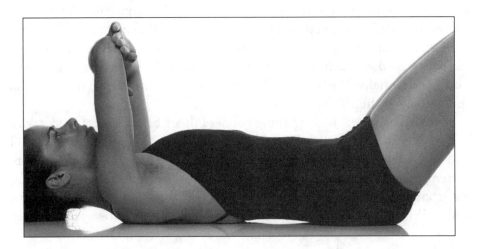

2. "Float" your waist and the back of your neck off the floor. The curves emphasized by this movement are the natural curves of the body. This is the neutral position. Many of us have been taught to flatten these curves by tucking or squeezing the buttocks, which is incorrect and unnatural.

### FUNDAMENTAL TWO: Breathing

This technique will make using your abdominals almost effortless.

1. Inhale and feel the back of the ribs spread wide on the floor.
2. Keeping the ribs wide, exhale and feel the abdominal muscles below the navel lift up and back as you imprint your spine.
3. Engage your abdominals into the spine and lengthen your body. Your abdominals should imprint into your spine. Imagine wearing a really tight one-piece swimsuit that flattens your belly.

### FUNDAMENTAL THREE: The Pelvic Bowl

The pelvic bowl is the triangle between your pubic bone and your hip bones.

1. Lying on your back in the neutral spine position, inhale and rock your pelvis forward. Your waist will rise higher off the floor, extending your spine.

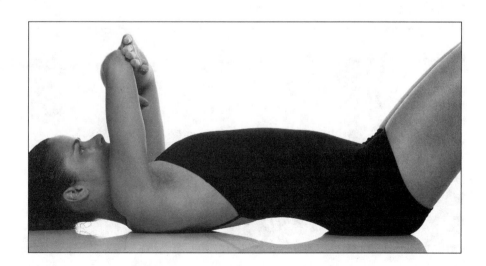

2. Exhale and rock backward until your waist is on the floor. The pelvis has moved into flexion. Do not use your legs, neck, hips, or any part of your anatomy other than your abdominals.

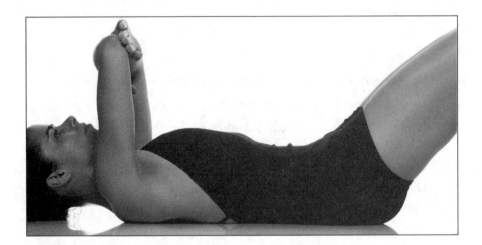

Besides using your pelvis in flexion and extension, you can also take it into rotation.

1. Rock your pelvis front to back, then side to side. Your abdominals initiate the rocking and rolling of the pelvis on the floor.

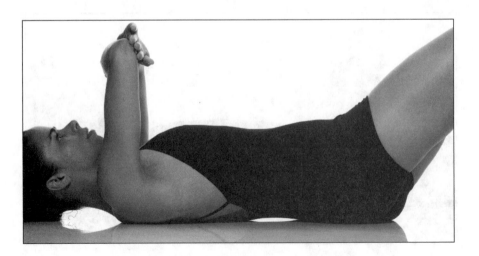

2. To rock to the left side, imprint the abdominals on your left side—the *obliques*—just below the navel. This will create a small movement of the pelvis swaying to the left.

3. Activate the right obliques below the navel to bring the pelvis back to the neutral spine position, then sway to the right. Don't use your legs and hips.

4. Circle your pelvis on the floor using your abdominals only. Imprint sequentially each part: tail, side, back, side. First clockwise, then counterclockwise. Use only your abdominals.

## Leg Fundamentals

Leg Fundamentals teach you to move your legs while the rest of your body stays still. Each movement isolates a different muscle and they all share the concepts detailed below.

### FUNDAMENTAL FOUR: The Knee Fold

The Knee Fold is an awareness exercise to learn to lift the legs from one of the deepest muscles of the body: the iliopsoas. The psoas connects our back lower ribs and crosses diagonally down the front of the pelvis to across the pubic bone, then attaches to the inner thigh bones. Visualize a string attached to the inner thigh being pulled up your spine to help lift your leg. The abdominals counterbalance the pull of the psoas. The abdominal muscles elongate and narrow. The pelvis remains in the neutral position. The abdominal muscles on the opposite side of your pelvis from the Knee Fold leg have to engage deeper or the pelvis will rock.

1. Lie on your back with your knees bent and feet flat on the floor. Your pelvis should be in the neutral position.

2. Place your left hand on the front of the hip where the thigh bones connect to the pelvis.

3. Place your right hand on your right knee. Fold the right knee up, with the abdominals moving back into the spine.

4. Rest the right foot back on the floor.

5. Switch hands. Repeat this movement with the left knee.

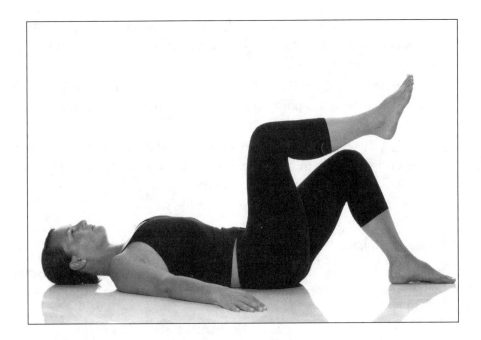

Here is a harder version:

1. Put your hands on either side of your navel. Press down to hollow your abdominals.

2. Fold your right knee up.

3. Lower your right knee and immediately fold the left one. Switch legs simultaneously; as one leg goes down, bring the other one up. This trains the abdominals to work deeply.

FUNDAMENTAL FIVE: The Knee Stir

1. Starting supine, feet on the floor, knees bent, fold your right knee and place your right hand on your lifted knee.

2. Circle the knee without moving your pelvis. If your pelvis stays still, you are using your obliques, which is the right connection.

3. Repeat with the other leg.

4. Now do this movement with both knees up, circling each knee in the same and then the opposite direction.

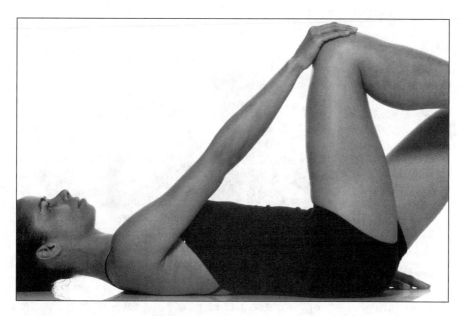

FUNDAMENTAL SIX: The Leg Slide

1. Slide your heel out to fully extend the leg, then slide your heel back toward the sitting bone.

2. Keep the pelvis stable throughout. Initiate the movement by activating the hamstrings, then allow gravity to pull the thigh to the floor.

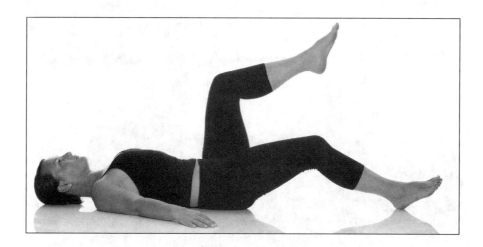

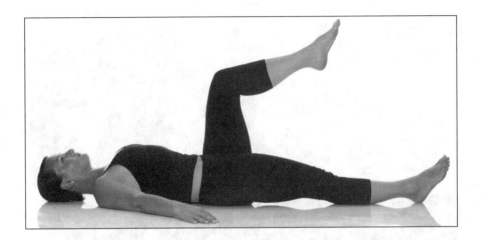

3.  Try simultaneously lengthening the right leg into a leg slide as the left leg goes into a Knee Fold. Switch simultaneously. Did your belly bulge out? If so, put your hands on the front of the pelvis to encourage the abs to lift and become hollow.

FUNDAMENTAL SEVEN: The Knee Sway

1.  Fold both bent legs up off the floor with your arms folded above your chest.

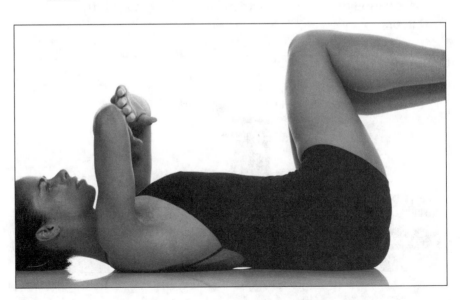

2. Sway your knees to the right without touching the floor; the left side of your pelvis will rock off the floor.

3. Sway both knees to the right. Use your left obliques to bring your pelvis back to the neutral position.

4. Repeat several times.

### FUNDAMENTAL EIGHT: Bridging

Now that you know how to use your legs and your torso, combine them in an active movement.

1. Imagine your feet have four corners: two on either side of the ball of the foot and two on the heel. With equal pressure on the four points, lift your hips up. Your knees should be parallel and in line with your feet. Don't allow your abs to bulge out. Your sitting bones should move closer to your heels and your knees should be over your feet.

2. Lower your entire spine in one movement. The highest point in the bridge should be your hip bones.

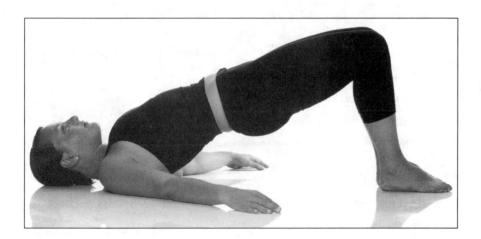

Here is a harder version:

1. Lift your pelvis up.

2. Knee fold your right leg.

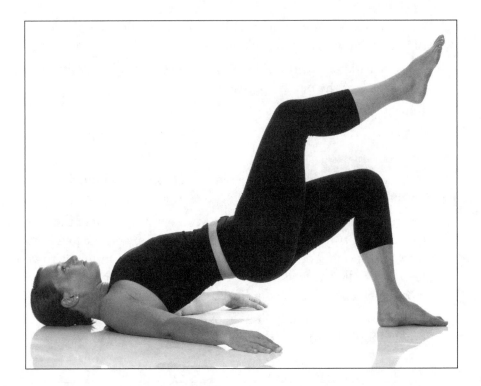

3. Return your right foot to the floor, but keep your hips level in a bridge.

4. Lift your left leg into a Knee Fold.

5. Return the left foot to the floor.

6. Return the hips to the floor.

## The Head Fundamental

The Head Fundamental is a spinal movement that elongates the neck and supports the head.

### FUNDAMENTAL NINE: The Head Float

The Head Float is a spinal movement to raise the head.

1. Lie on the floor in the neutral spine position with your knees bent and your feet flat on the floor.

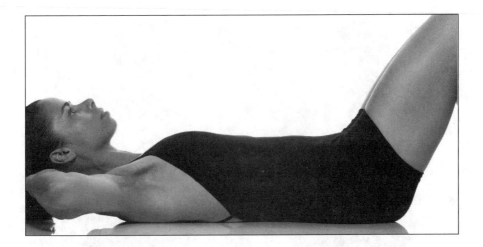

2. Bring your arms up and lace your hands behind your head. Let your head ride in your hands to float your head off the floor. Keep your neck long and don't tuck in your chin. Imagine someone is behind you supporting the weight of your head and gently stretching your neck so that it becomes longer.

3. To lift your head higher, your spine must do the rest. Sink your front ribs to your back ribs and curl forward.

4. Lengthen the back of the spine to return to the floor. Try to do this with your hands by your sides.

## The Arm Fundamentals

The Arm Fundamentals teach us that our shoulders have "arms" that begin midback.

### FUNDAMENTAL TEN: Rib Cage Arms

The point of this movement is to remind you that your arms start at your shoulder blades, or scapulae. The arms are meant to work from muscles around the scapulae and the back to reduce the shoulders' workload. The shoulder blade is a lever that lifts the arm bones.

1. Lie with your arms by your side. (The photos on the following page show the back.) You should feel width across your shoulders front and back.

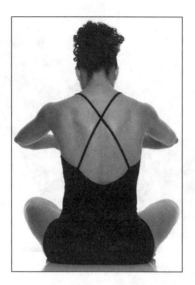 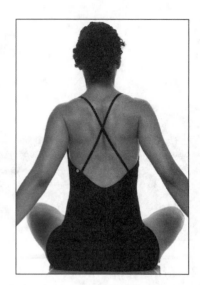

2. Imagine your shoulder blades are windshield wipers. Glide the scapulae (shoulder blades) wide on the ribs to move the arms on the floor to shoulder height, then over your head if possible. Your entire arm, the windshield wiper, should be cleaning the floor. The tip of each scapula should widen to the side of your ribs.

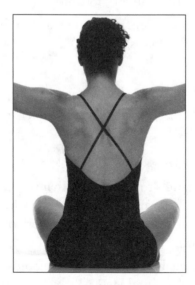

3. Return the arms to your sides.

FUNDAMENTAL ELEVEN: Arm Circles

1. Lie on your back with your arms at your sides, palms facing your hips.

2. Lift your hands to the ceiling directly above your shoulders. Feel the head of the arm bone settle into its socket.

3. As you lower your arms overhead, feel the glide of your shoulder blades. Your ribs should remain soft and wide on the floor.

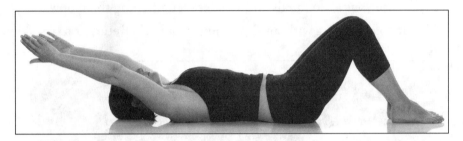

4. Slide your arms on the floor in a circular motion to shoulder height.

5. Windshield wipe your arms back to the sides of your hips. Your arms from shoulder height are gradually rotating inward with the palms facing the hips. Keep the front and the back of the shoulders wide.

6. Reverse the circle.

## Front Fundamentals

Front Fundamentals activate your back.

FUNDAMENTAL TWELVE: Flight

1. Lie on your belly with your arms at your sides.

2. Lift your abdominals and reach your fingers toward your toes.

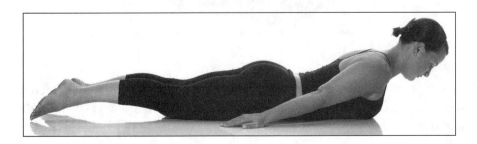

3. Lengthen your torso and keep your neck long.

4. Engage your back muscles and lift your sternum off the floor. Do not let your lower back collapse.

FUNDAMENTAL THIRTEEN: Hip Extension

1. Lie on your belly with your head resting on your arms.

2. Engage your abdominals and visualize lengthening them upward.

3. Lift your right leg without shortening your back. Return it to the floor.

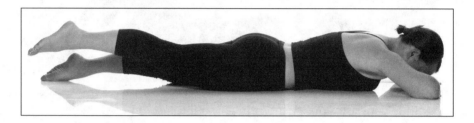

4. Repeat with your left leg.

Here is a harder version:

1. Extend your arms in front of you in the shape of the letter V.

2. Imagine you have two additional limbs—the head and the tailbone—lengthening away from your belly button.

3. Lift both legs and arms off the floor. Float.

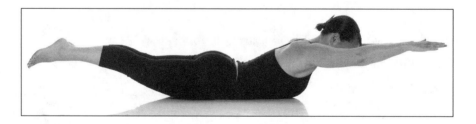

FUNDAMENTAL FOURTEEN: The Cat

The Cat is a spinal movement for flexion and extension on all fours. You need this movement now because your lower back should be rounded (flexed) after the Extension Fundamentals.

1. Lift up to all fours with your weight on your hands and knees. Feel your spine in its natural curves.

2. Connect your shoulder blades to hug around the sides of your ribs.

3. Imprint the abdominals into your spine to curve it upward like a scared cat. This is flexion of the spine.

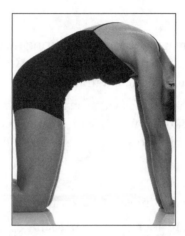

4. Reverse this curve by lifting your head and tail up.

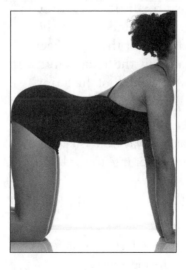

5. Return to the neutral spine position.

# The Foundations

The Foundations are the Standing Fundamentals: a higher level of information to create awareness in complex movements.

## Foundation One

### The Pelvic Foundation

1. Stand tall and imagine that you are lifting the pelvic floor—draw up, lift, and slightly squeeze the small space between the coccyx bone (in back) and the pubic bone (in front).

2. Inhale, then exhale to activate the *transversus muscle* by pulling in to lift your belly button, which will create a concavity beneath your navel. This will help you access the deepest abdominals.

### The Standing Foundation

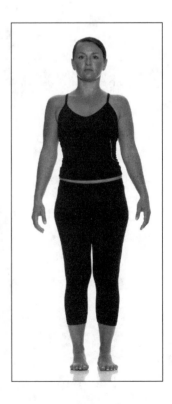

1. Stand with your feet in parallel position.

2. Imagine there are four points on each foot. The first two are on either side of the ball of your foot: one near the big toe and the other near the little toe. At the back of the foot, the points are on the inside and the outside of the heel. Feel the weight equally on the four points. Feel the arches of your foot like tiny domes.

3. Connect the pelvis over the feet, with your rib cage floating away from the waist and the head lengthening toward the ceiling.

4. Rock onto your heels, then onto the balls of your feet.

5. Shift to the outside edges of the feet, then roll onto the inside edges.

6. Return to the neutral position. Exhale.

7. Bend your knees and hinge into a squat. Inhale. Place one hand on your navel and the other hand on your lower back. Feel equal length front and back.

8. Put both of your hands in front where the thigh bone connects to the pelvis. Feel a nice fold in front of the hips.

9. Exhale and straighten your legs.

The Single-Leg Stance

1. Stand on one leg and rest the heel of the other foot on top of the standing foot.

2. Concentrate your weight on the outside hip of the standing leg. This will feel as if you are sitting into your hip, but be sure the shift is sideways, not to the back.

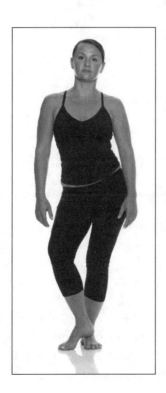

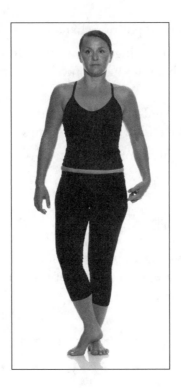

3. Use the outside muscles of the thighs to move back to the start position. The hips become level when activating these muscles.

4. Repeat on the other side.

## Foundation Two: The Domes

There are four domes. The main one is the pelvic dome. The pelvis is the
linchpin that connects the spine to the legs. The bottom of the pelvis consists
of four points (just like the foot). The sitting bones are at the bottom of the
back of the pelvis. The front of the pelvis is the pubis, which we divide into a
left and a right side. Connecting to these four points are the muscles of the
pelvic floor. Imagine they are like a dome within the pelvic bones. Imagine lifting up this pelvic dome like an elevator; this will naturally and easily activate
the abdominals. Your deepest abdominal, the transversus, attaches to your
diaphragm, which is your second dome. It is the oxygen pump. Pretend that

the diaphragm is a parachute. On the inhale the parachute descends down in the rib cage. On the exhale it floats up in the rib cage. The third dome is in the roof of your mouth, where your spine ends inside of your skull. The fourth dome is the arches of your feet. Now that you know where all these domes are located, try this exercise:

1. Stand with your feet in parallel position.

2. Imagine bringing the four domes to suspend over each other.

3. Inhale, then exhale, lifting the arch dome of the foot; the pelvic floor dome; the diaphragm dome; and the roof dome. Feel how your spine lengthens and the muscles of your legs activate when these domes lift up.

Now try this exercise while bending and straightening the legs. Inhale upon standing; exhale while bending the knees. Inhale in bent knee position; exhale and lift the domes as you straighten your legs.

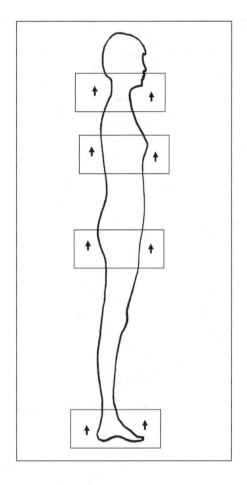

## Foundation Three: The Bow

The Bow teaches you to flex your upper spine forward but keep your lower body and legs stable. The Bow is a lengthened forward flexion that avoids cervical compression.

1. Stand with your feet in parallel position and your hands in prayer position against your breastbone.

2. Use your hands to help soften your breastbone to bow your upper spine. This is to help open the back ribs and the space between your shoulder blades. Your weight still remains over your feet and pelvic foundation. Do not allow the rib cage to move forward.

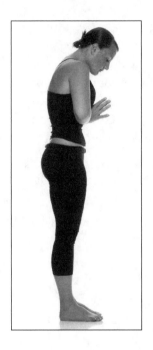

## Foundation Four: Spinal Arms

There are three versions of Spinal Arms.

### Version 1

1. Place your hands on your thighs in the front where they connect to your spine.

2. Lift your breastbone to the ceiling. Your head follows the spine in extension. Make your legs work.

3. Lengthen your spine in front and back and lift all four domes.

### Version 2

1. Reach both your arms above your head in the shape of the letter V.

2. Lengthen your left side with your left arm

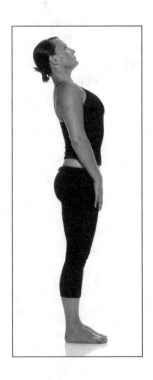

reaching up to the ceiling. Your spine will bend to the side in the shape of the letter C.

3. Return to the Standing Foundation by lengthening the right side to match the new length of the left side. Your arms are doing nothing; they get a free ride from the spinal movement.

4. Reach your right arm to the ceiling and bend your spine to the left, creating a reverse C.

5. Return to the Standing Foundation. Your weight remains on both legs.

Version 3

1. Fold your arms in front of you at shoulder height. Your forearms are placed on top of each other in the *I Dream of Jeannie* position.

2. Twist your upper spine and keep your hips facing front. The rib cage dome is like a lazy Susan—a disk that rotates. The rotation of the rib cage dome is suspended above the pelvic dome and the arch dome of the foot.

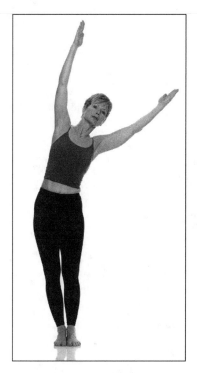

This is a lot of information, and you may be overwhelmed. Relax and reread this chapter a few times. You will see that these positions are minimovements for all the parts of your body that start at the center and move outward. They are to teach you to move more easily and efficiently.

We can all be lazy; we try to move in parts and avoid using the entire body. For daily tasks we move from the periphery and not from the core. If we are on the tennis court, we may put our entire body into the swing because we have been taught that this is how the pros do it. This is true because they are naturally smart movers. They do not "save" their energy even when they do everyday motions. They use deeper muscles—those closer to the bone. Gradually you will do this, too.

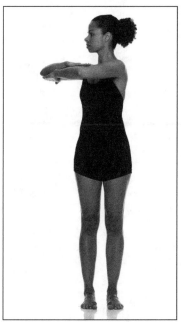

# The Classical Mat

Once these Classical Pilates mat exercises were considered too difficult for nondancers. Now they are a standard. Don't take them for granted, though. Remember, the Pilates philosophy is quality, not quantity. You can always go deeper.

Each of the following exercises leads to the next one, so you have a short full-body routine that you can sequence into a flowing workout. If you learn these exercises, the cues and the movement, the physical and the mind, are combined into a functional workout.

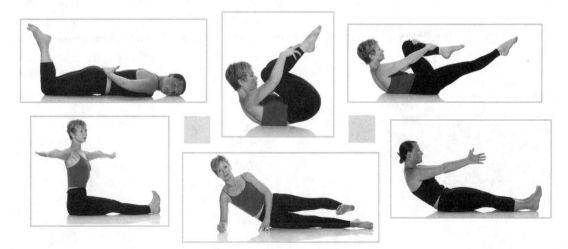

# SINGLE-LEG STRETCH

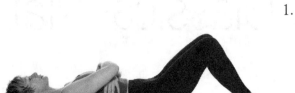

## To Start

1. Lie on your back in the neutral spine position with your feet on the floor and knees up and arms crossed on your rib cage. Inhale and bellow your back ribs into the floor. Exhale and deepen the abs in and up. Picture the pelvic dome imprinting your *sacrum* wider and longer on the floor. The pelvic dome lifts up and softens your lower ribs deeper into the floor.

2. Inhale and on the next exhale, with this abdominal connection, lift your right knee up to practice the Knee Fold fundamental.

3. Inhale, then on the next exhale, knee fold the left knee up.

4. Inhale and float your head up, exhale, then bow the thoracic spine by deepening the abdominals into the spine. With the Bow in this supine position, you can observe your pelvis and the abdominal muscles moving in and up at all times.

5. Inhale and place your left hand on your right knee and your right hand on your right ankle as you extend your left leg out in front of you. Your lower back at your waist should not arch off the floor.

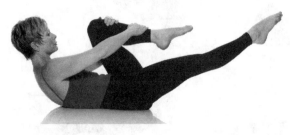

The pelvis is in neutral. The triangle of the points of your pubis bone and your two hip bones should be like the flat surface of a table.

## The Movement

6. On the exhale, switch legs and hands.

7. Inhale and switch again.

8. Sink the front of the pelvis deeper with every switch of the leg. You are bowing to your hollowed abdominals. Focus forward and stay lifted in the upper body. Keep your elbows high. Repeat five to ten sets.

9. At the end of your sets, lower your straight leg down on the floor and slide your folded knee next to it. Press both legs down into the floor as you extend your spine and arms overhead to begin the Roll-Up.

## Technique

Imagine the pelvic triangle—the triangle from the pubis to both hip bones—is a weight that is attached to the floor. With every switch, there is a counterreach, an opposition, where the spine lengthens more as the legs reach in the opposite direction.

## Goals

The spine remains stabilized throughout the exercise. There should not be any rocking of the pelvis when switching the legs.

## Modifications

For beginners, extend the leg to the ceiling. If you feel a pull in your back, it is a sign that you are not using your abdominals deeply.

## Variations

When the movement becomes easier, lower the leg closer to the floor.

# II ROLL-UP

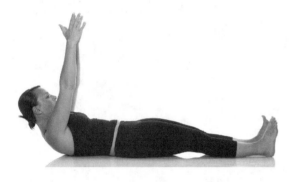

## To Start

1. Lie on your back, arms overhead, legs lengthened and together, and feet flexed.

2. Inhale and lift your arms from your shoulder blades toward the ceiling with your palms facing each other.

### The Movement

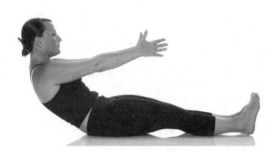

3. Begin bowing on the exhale as you reach toward your feet. Peel your flexed spine off the floor until you are sitting on your pelvis with your arms reaching forward. You should feel the shoulder blades wrapping around your ribs. There is space between your ears and your shoulders because you are moving your arms from your scapulae.

4. Inhale, feel your back ribs widen as you pelvic tilt to initiate the Roll-Down.

5. Exhale and deepen the abdominals in toward the sacrum. These inward movements of the abdominals facilitate your rolling down. Roll down by carefully placing each spinal vertebra on the floor one by one. Once your head is back on the floor, raise your arms overhead from your scapulae. When you imprint the front body into the back body, the spine lengthens.

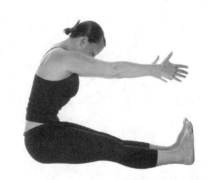

6. Repeat three to five times.

7. To end, bring your arms to the ceiling and float your head up; exhale and roll up to sitting. Double knee fold while you rock back on your tailbone. Grasp your knees with your arms and round your back.

## Technique

Imagine your spine and legs are like Velcro. As you roll up, feel your spine unfasten from the floor. On the Roll-Down, the front body deepens into the spine to help Velcro the spine longer on the floor. Keep the legs glued to the floor with the Velcro image. When you're lying on the floor with your arms overhead and legs straight, the lumbar spine (waist) and cervical spine (neck) can return to their natural curves; the action of rolling the spine on and off the floor flattens these curves.

## Goals

The Roll-Up enhances deep core strengthening and spinal articulation. This is great for discovering new spaces between the vertebrae of your spine.

## Modifications

If your back and leg muscles are tight, bend your knees. Also, place your feet under a low sofa to anchor your body.

## Variations

Slow the speed of the movement to eliminate momentum.

# ||| ROLLING LIKE A BALL

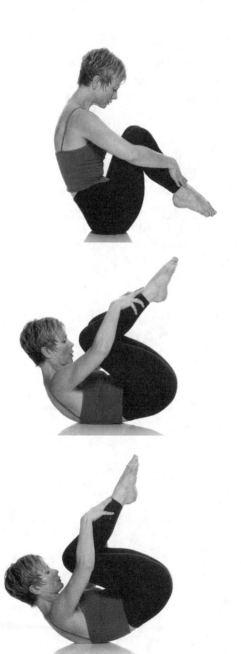

## To Start

1. Balance on your sitting bones, your hands resting on your knees or shins; your back is rounded. You want to bring your spine into the shape of a C. Your arms are creating the shape of a ball with your elbows extended outward.

2. Suspend in this position and practice the breath pattern to deepen the use of your abdominals. Inhale and feel the back widen and release more with a rounded spine like the shape of a ball. Exhale and watch your center sink toward your spine. Each breath should deepen the back in the shape of a ball. The breath should not distort the ball shape of the body.

## The Movement

3. Inhale and balance. Exhale while maintaining the ball shape and lifting your pelvic dome to initiate a roll backward and inhale to roll to the shoulder blades. Do not throw the head backward. The movement begins from your pelvic sphere.

4. Immediately exhale quickly to roll back to the suspended position.

5. Repeat three more sets.

6. Inhale and then exhale, and release your legs to come to sitting up, legs extended and arms at the sides at shoulder height.

## Technique

Do not allow momentum to drive the exercise. Initiate the movement from the pelvic bowl. Do not flip your head or legs.

## Goals

This exercise teaches you to flex your back while maintaining abdominal control. How you maintain the movement will determine its fluidity.

## Modifications

The most important part of this exercise is learning to round the spine and maintain abdominal control. Hold your knees farther away from your body if necessary.

## Variations

Pull your knees in close to your body by wrapping your arms tighter.

# IV  SPINE TWIST

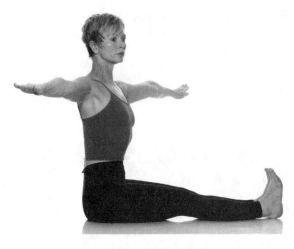

## To Start

1. Sit up tall on your sitting bones with your legs straight out and your arms at shoulder height suspended to each side. Imagine your fingertips reaching to the side walls.

2. Your legs are actively lengthening to the front of the room with your feet flexed. Just as in the standing foundation, you activate the quadriceps to lift the kneecaps as you press the back of your legs into the floor.

3. Dome your pelvic floor up and feel how it lifts the ribs. The ribs need to lengthen equally away from the pelvis. This is very important for rotation of the spine.

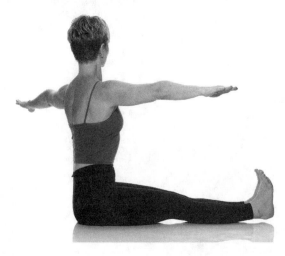

## The Movement

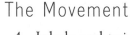

4. Inhale and twist your spine to the left. Your arms feel like they are riding on top of the rotating ribs. The shoulder blades stay wide and stable on the back ribs during the movement.

5. Exhale, reactivating the pelvic dome and the rib cage dome to return your ribs to face front. Remember the diaphragm rises inside the rib cage on the exhale. The arms remain suspended to each side at shoulder height.

6. Inhale, lengthen, and rotate your spine to the right with your arms at shoulder height.

7. Exhale, lift the pelvic floor and abdominals, and return your torso to face front.

8. Repeat three sets.

9. To end, inhale and twist your spine to the left. Reach your left hand to the floor behind you. Slide the left side of your spine onto the floor. You are now lying on your left side with both legs straight and slightly in front of you. Your right hand is on the floor near your lower ribs with your elbow pointing to the ceiling.

## Technique

Imagine your spine is like a spiral staircase. As you rotate, the steps are at equal distance from each other. Or imagine your spine like the barbershop pole with the red stripe. The barbershop pole is turning, which gives the illusion of the stripe spiraling up. This is your spine twisting. In a slumped posture you lose the head/tail connection. The result is that your head rotates but your spine stays behind.

## Goals

Visualize the rib cage as a sphere turning above the larger sphere of the pelvis. The spheres are suspended and floating above each other equally. The breath and the diaphragm help you to find new volume in your rib cage and more movement. Rotation of the rib cage is very important for daily tasks.

## Modifications

If you are unable to sit up with a neutral spine, sit on a prop such as a towel or pillow. Make sure the prop is high enough to allow you to sit evenly on the sitting bones in the back and to feel as if your pubic bone can touch the floor in the front. If your hamstrings are tight, bend your knees.

## Variations

Add a pulse at the end of each rotation before returning to the center.

# V SIDE KICK

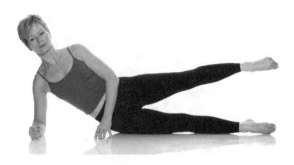

## To Start

1. Lie on your side with your legs extended parallel and in a 45-degree angle in front of your hips. Support your upper body weight on your forearm with your other hand in front of your waist on the floor.

2. Your spine is in the neutral position. Your head is aligned over your rib cage, which is over your pelvis. Lift your waist higher off the floor by pressing firmly down on your forearm.

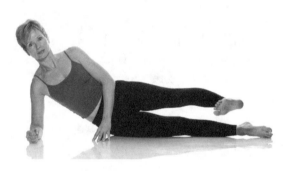

3. Practice lifting the abdominals without changing the length of your neutral spine. Inhale and widen the lower ribs. Exhale and engage the pelvic dome lift as the diaphragm rises in your ribs.

4. Lift the top leg up, keeping the pelvis calm. Imagine you are balancing champagne glasses on this leg.

## The Movement

5. Inhale and slowly swing the leg forward with a flexed foot, maintaining the equal distance of the pelvis and the rib cage.

6. Exhale and give a double pulse forward.

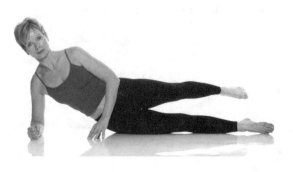

7. Swing your top leg backward with a pointed foot. Allow the front of the hip to be long while engaging your pelvic center during the entire movement. Maintain length between your pelvis

and rib cage. The top hip should always be in the same line as the bottom hip.

8. Repeat eight full leg swings forward and backward.

9. To roll to the other side, extend your entire body on your side with both arms reaching over your head. Try to distribute your weight throughout your entire body. This may be hard to do but it is very important. Try to keep your legs and arms suspended off the floor. Roll onto your back, then to your other side. Can you roll in one piece?

10. Repeat the leg swing sequence on this other side.

11. To end, roll your entire body as one piece onto your belly.

## Technique

Imagine the top of your head has puppet strings that pull you in one direction while your tailbone and legs are being pulled in the opposite direction from your center.

## Goals

This exercise teaches torso stability combined with mobility of the legs. Notice how you need to use your abdominals differently when the leg swings forward as compared to backward. When you swing the leg forward, your abs have to sink deeper to prevent the top hip from moving forward with the leg. As you swing the leg backward in extension, you need to move the abdominals upward to prevent the top hip from rolling backward, or even worse, from hyperextending the back.

## Modifications

Bend your bottom leg for a more secure base. Reduce the leg swing if your hamstrings are tight.

## Variations

Align legs in a straight line to your spine.

# VI  DOUBLE-LEG KICK

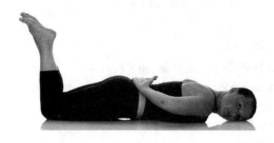

## To Start

1. Lying face down, with your head turned so the cheek rests on its side, interlock your hands behind your back. Your bent elbows can rest on your sides. Your knees are bent and together.

2. Inhale and on the exhale, practice engaging the pelvic dome. The floor gives you tremendous information. You can allow your body to sink in or you can lift your navel off the floor and anchor your pelvic triangle on the floor. Feel how the pelvic triangle lifts off the floor, which helps you to lengthen. You should feel longer on the floor when you engage your abdominals.

## The Movement

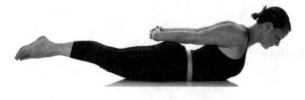

3. Exhale and pulse your lower legs with flexed feet three times. You should feel a long line on the floor from the top of your front hips to the knees. Do not let the hips flex.

4. With your arms and legs extended, inhale and extend your spine and head, and bring your shoulder blades together. Imagine you are the bow of a ship pressing through the waves. Were you able to feel the front of the hips and thighs stay elongated throughout the movement?

5. Exhale and return the spine to the floor while softening the elbows to the sides of your body. Simultaneously pulse your bent knees with flexed feet three times.

6. Repeat three sets.

7. Rest by pushing up to the Cat Fundamental in the "scared" position.

## Technique

Imagine you have two conveyor belts under your body. One starts at your waist to lengthen your ribs and head away from your pelvis. The other one at the waist also moves the pelvis and legs away from the top of your head. If you crunch your abdominals, notice it will not allow your body to comfortably move in extension.

## Goals

This exercise strengthens the back of the body while maintaining length. Extension exercises are the counterpoint to forward flexion from endless sitting.

## Modifications

If you have knee problems, make the bending and the pulsing of the knees smaller and slower. If your back is weak, limit your range of motion. Keep the abdominal connection at all times.

1. Practice pulling your shoulder blades together with the arms straight and lifting the upper spine up to a comfortable range for you. The flight fundamental is the motion.

2. Slowly bend your knees with legs parallel to each other. Keep the spine long. Place your hands on your buttocks and lengthen them away from the top of the head. The legs are doing the work. Don't allow the movement to crunch in your lower back.

41

# DOUBLE-LEG KICK
*(continued)*

3. Lift one leg up at a time.
4. Lift both legs up.

## Variations
Keep the legs off the floor the entire time, bent or straight.

# 5

# Being Vertical

I remember visiting a Pilates studio and watching a trainer correct a client's posture of rounded upper back, forward head, and tucked pelvis. But when the client, a man in his fifties, rose to stand from the supine position, I saw his "old" postural habit reappear. The corrections were *lost in translation* to the upright position!

Standing Pilates was developed to teach correct alignment in functional positions. The floor exercises were reconfigured to standing on both legs and then transferring the weight to one leg. These exercises have been quickly adopted because they are interesting and beneficial, particularly for the aging population. For instance, osteoporosis prevention requires weight-bearing exercise (for more on osteoporosis, refer to appendix B). Previously, such exercises were minimal in the Pilates repertoire. Another problem Standing Pilates can prevent is prolapse, which is the result of a weakened pelvic floor.

Standing Pilates promotes the well-being of the pelvic floor because its engagement is crucial to performing the exercises. The pelvic floor performs three functions:

1. *Supportive:* to maintain the position of internal organs. We use the pelvic floor when we cough, laugh, or sneeze. Because these actions

create internal abdominal pressure, the pelvic floor responds by keeping everything in line. If the pelvic floor is weak, however, the contents of the pelvis (or the internal organs) can prolapse, or fall.

2. *Sphincteric:* to prevent incontinence. Twenty-five million Americans suffer from this problem.

3. *Sexual:* to increase sexual stimulation. Women who exercise the pelvic floor muscles report enhanced sexual feeling.

The pelvic floor can be compromised or damaged from childbirth, surgery (prostectomy for men and hysterectomy for women), postmenopausal estrogen deficiency, diabetes, multiple sclerosis, smokers' cough, and obesity.

The pelvic floor needs to be engaged during standing exercise. The pelvic floor muscles, the multifidus, the diaphragm, and the transversus abdominus form a cylinder, or a support, for the spine. These muscles work together in maintaining intraabdominal pressure, which is needed to release pressure from the spine and to support internal organs during exertion.

Standing Pilates is full-body exercise that requires us to focus on how the body moves and reacts in order to balance. Practice leads to a neurorepatterning that will translate into functional, correct movement in standing, sitting, or bending over to pick up something.

How does Standing Pilates compare with the Classical Mat? They are both full-body exercises, but standing adds more "real estate" to the equation. In general, Standing Pilates is easier to do if you are not terribly flexible, but it demands more brain activity because of the balance element. Most clients now do some of each.

## Mirrors: Standing's Secret Tool

You already know that Pilates depends on proper form. It is controlled, concentrated, and centered exercise. You need to continuously check your positions. If you are working with a Pilates trainer, this person will check, too. The hope is that this method gets into your body and becomes internal. Alignment is key to working the muscles in a balanced condition. When a joint is poorly aligned, certain muscles are working more and others are becoming deconditioned.

One of the best things about Standing Pilates is that you can see yourself. When you are lying on your back, it is hard to see your body's reflection. Mirrors have been a secret tool in helping me to change my body so that it is better both functionally and aesthetically. I have mirrors everywhere: by my desk, next to my dining table, in my dressing area. As I walk on the streets in New York, I can see my posture in the shop windows.

Visual cues are a tool for body change. Are you aware when you are sitting with your legs crossed and your spine slumped for thirty minutes? Unless a trainer reminds you to change your position or realign your spine, you need to be constantly on task. To develop a smart body, awareness is key.

Use the mirror as an awareness tool. Try to suspend judgment about your thighs or chest, or whatever. Start at the feet. Are you concentrating your weight on the inside of your feet or the outside? Are your feet parallel or turned out? Look at the ankle joints. Are the ankles aligned over the toes? Is the distance from the inside/outside of the ankles the same from the floor? Are the knees aligned over the ankles? Are the hips level? Is one hip more forward than the other? Stand on one leg. How does the alignment of the leg change? Imagine a plumb line going through the bones. Imagine your spine as different-size spheres suspended over each other. Is your pelvic sphere over your feet, rib cage sphere over the pelvis, and head sphere over the other two spheres?

Observe how the fabric of your clothes drapes over your body. Slump, and observe how there are more wrinkles. Stand with more weight on one leg, observing how the clothing is different on one leg than the other. With good posture, the clothes hang better.

## Watching Others, Watching Yourself

Once you are accustomed to looking at your body, start looking at others, particularly those with similar shapes. Notice how they move. How does poor body alignment affect a person's walk? When you are in a movie theater, notice how people sit for two hours with crossed legs and do not change position— not even to alternate the crossed leg position!

Smart bodies change position frequently. Some really smart movers are ambidextrous. These lucky people feel the need for movement. You need to schedule position changes to energize your body while it is awake.

Observe how you and others eat. How much food do you eat? How quickly do you eat? The issue is eating too much, too fast. Quantity reduction, not food manipulation, is the Pilates approach to weight loss. Not nutrient manipulation. Just eating less and finding quality time to eat.

Begin paying attention and making changes gradually and consistently. The Fundamentals and the Foundations are the minimovements that train the brain to move the body correctly. When you are awake, be aware; this combination will result in an energetic body.

## Pilates Takes a Stance

There are twenty-two standing exercises, and each has three levels. Level I is a preparation position that helps you to organize your body parts. Practice near a wall for support if needed. You will need a mirror so that you can check your position. If you are unsteady, start your practice wearing athletic shoes.

Level II is the actual exercise that will build strength, balance, and coordination skills with the suggested repetitions. Level III is complex movement. For very advanced movers, there are additional variations that are even more challenging. You can mix these levels in any way you choose. You can start at Level I and continue to Level II, then III. If you do all three levels, reduce the number of reps per level so that you do not exhaust yourself.

However, you may be at Level I for some exercises, Level II for others, and even Level III for a few, depending on your balance, flexibility, and coordination. At any stage, you may test yourself by trying to do one of the movements with your eyes closed. Proprioception—awareness of where your body is in space—will decrease by 30 percent when you close your eyes. You may have to drop a level or decrease the repetitions because your brain will have to work that much harder. To move your body, your brain is working to balance on one leg and move from one spatial plane to two or more; change the spine from flexion to extension; increase the range of motion; add length by extending a limb or two away from your center. Focus is critical for these exercises.

Standing Pilates is an exercise sequence that requires conscious breathing. Every movement is initiated by an inhalation or an exhalation. If you are a novice, don't worry if you inhaled when you should have exhaled. In general, if you exhale during flexion, the movement is easier. But other than ease, it won't matter if you get mixed up. Just don't hold your breath. Conscious rhythmic breathing is a challenge. Ultimately, it is a pleasure.

A true Pilates progression is a layering of movement that requires total focus so that the information from your brain gets to your body. This process is continuous, improving your body and your brain. Once you learn to pay attention, you won't stop, because making these connections is interesting and it works. Bodies can improve functionally and aesthetically. Smart exercise is the fastest way to get the body you want.

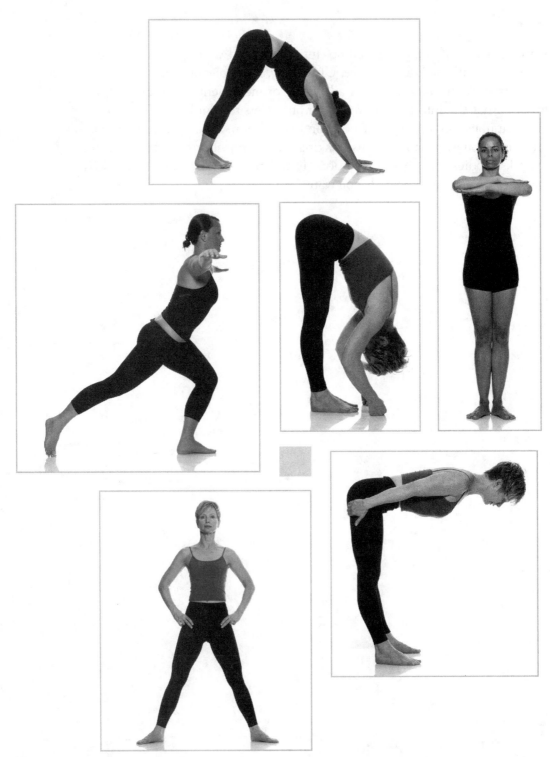

# 6

# The Standing Exercises

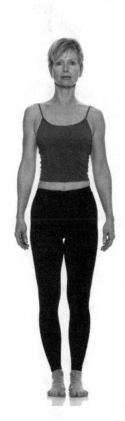

L earn the standing exercises by following the description of the choreography and looking at the photos. There is a pattern to all the Standing sequences:

1. You start in the Standing Foundation, or with your legs close as in Pilates first position or farther apart at hip distance.

2. You begin with an inhale, then exhale for the next step, and so on for each step.

3. Level I is the preparation position.

4. Level II adds one or two elements.

5. Level III adds more movements and a lot of challenge.

Once you understand the sequence similarities, you can concentrate on the choreography, which is not complicated, and the form, which is always the same. Incorporating both the choreography and the form is the challenge.

The choreography comprises the steps in an exercise. Learning choreography develops movement memory and better coordination.

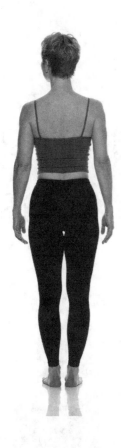

The form is the application of the Fundamentals and the Foundations. What does this mean?

- The Standing Foundation is your best posture with legs active, feet using all four corners, torso lengthened, and domes lifted on the exhalation.
- In the Pelvic Foundation the lift of the pelvic floor and the breathing technique enable your abdominals to activate fully and easily.
- The Bow is a lengthened forward flexion from the upper body. Flex your upper spine with the focus at the thoracic (around the bra line); minimize cervical flexion (neck), which most people tend to overflex; do not flex at all from the lumbar.
- The Knee Fold technique means that your leg lift will not distort your spine or hike up your hip.
- The Leg Slide means that when you extend your leg, you will not change the position of your hips.
- The Single-Leg Foundation means that when you shift onto one leg, you maintain alignment and do not sit into your hip or move backward.
- The Arms Fundamentals and Foundations reinforce that your arms move from your back.
- Conscious inhalation and exhalation ties everything together and assists focus, concentration, and effort.

To assist your body, think about what you want to happen using language that will trigger the response. Important words are:

| | | |
|---|---|---|
| engage | lengthen | initiate |
| sequence | narrow | float |
| activate | connect | lift |
| articulate | reach | extend |
| hollow | imprint | suspend |

Remember to listen, breathe, focus, and be aware, alive, and alert so that you are physical, neutral, parallel, and easeful. Avoid compressing, collapsing, pushing, tucking, grabbing, dragging, clenching, and performing mindless motion.

Think of your torso as a lengthened rectangle that you maintain as your arms and legs move in various directions. You can see in the mirror how well you are keeping it all together. If you start to lose it, back up, and go smaller or lower, or closer or slower. Remember that you are standing, squatting, bending, kneeling, lifting, twisting, and extending. These are functional actions you do every day. The difference is that you are *paying attention to them* while you do them. And even when this form gets into your muscle memory, you will still want to pay attention. Because moving well will become a pleasure.

# 1   THE HUNDRED

Forward Flexion and Breathing

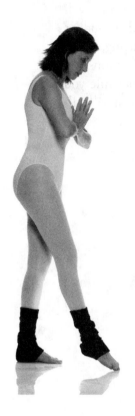

## Level 1

Preparation

1. Inhale in the Standing Foundation.

2. Exhale and press your palms together in prayer position in line with your breastbone with elbows out to the side.

3. Inhale, connect your feet to the ground, and activate your legs. The inner thighs wrap back.

4. Exhale and bow over your prayer hands. The ribs stay lifted up away from the hips.

5. Inhale, feel the back of the ribs widen, and lift your back rib cage toward the ceiling. (The ribs move into the body, back, and up.)

6. Exhale, engage the lower abdominals (pelvic floor), and glide your right pointed foot forward along the floor.

7. Inhale for four long counts.

8. Exhale for six counts while you lift up your abdominals, breathing into the back of your ribs.

9. Repeat steps 7 and 8 five times (fifty counts total). Keep the standing leg and torso active and energy out through the front leg. Your weight is distributed from your feet to the top of your head with your torso "centered" over the supporting leg.

10. Inhale to return to the Standing Foundation. Refocus your eyes in the mirror.

11. Repeat on the left leg.

## Level II

Adds a leg lift and an arm beat.

1. Inhale in the Standing Foundation with arms by your sides and fingers reaching to the floor.

2. Exhale, bow, and lift up your right pointed foot about three inches.

3. Inhale and beat your arms back four counts; exhale for six beats. Repeat this set five times for a total count of fifty.

4. Inhale while unbowing your upper spine to the Standing Foundation on both feet.

5. Exhale and shift to the right foot.

6. Repeat on the left leg.

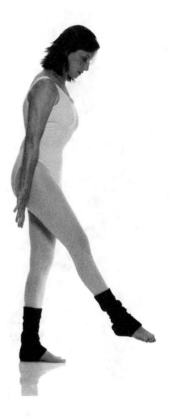

# THE HUNDRED

*(continued)*

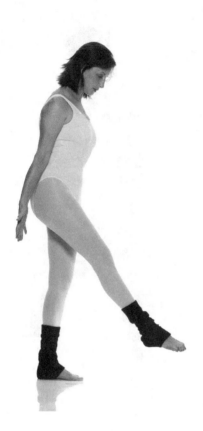

## Level III

Adds a higher leg lift and arm rotation with the beats.

1. Inhale in the Standing Foundation with arms by your sides.

2. Exhale, bow, and lift your right pointed foot about five inches off the floor.

3. Inhale, rotate your arms inward (palms facing back), and beat for four counts.

4. Exhale while externally rotating the arms (palms facing forward) and beat for six counts. A set is a full breath, inhalation and exhalation, with arms moving; repeat for a total of five sets.

5. Inhale and return to the Standing Foundation and actively lengthen up with a straight spine.

6. Repeat on the left leg.

## Tall Technique

Pay attention to your feet. Lift up the arches so that you feel the inside and outside edges of each foot equally. Notice how really using your feet changes your posture and the muscularity of your legs.

In prayer position, can you equally press each finger and the heels of your hands together? Notice how pressing your hands together lifts the elbows out to the sides. Do you also feel how the tone under your armpits changes?

Shoulders are relaxed yet broad and strong. The shoulder blades are gently sliding down the back. The outside edges of the scapulae move closer to the armpits. These actions should widen the space between the shoulder blades. Notice how you feel new width in the front of your body as well as the back. Pay attention to your back and your front will follow.

Awareness of the combination of your feet and your hands working together changes the length of the lower and upper body. The feet are rooted strongly downward and the upper body is floating up from this new strength. The hands activate the upper body. Pay attention to the hands connected to the arms. Arm rotation starts in the shoulder socket that connects to the humerus bone in the top of the arm. If your feet and hands are lazy, it is harder to balance, which leads to incorrect compensations.

## Goals

Active, accurate breath pattern without any distortion of the body position. The breath warms up your body. Changing your focus challenges balance because vision gives you stability. When your focus is down at your feet, you must rearrange your perspective, and balancing becomes more challenging.

## Modifications

Those with osteoporosis can eliminate the bow.

## Variations

Small releves (heel raises) as you beat on each breath. Two releves during the inhale and two on the exhale. On "percussive" breathing, which is faster and with an emphatic exhale, inhale quickly and blow out the exhale.

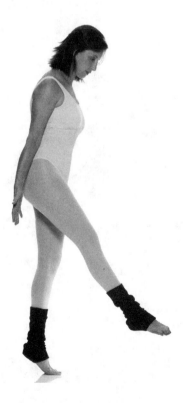

55

# 2 LEG CIRCLES

Pelvic Stability and Differentiation at the Hip.

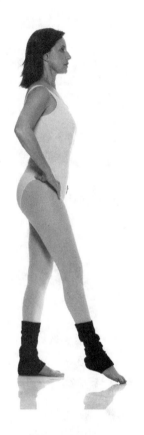

## Level I

Preparation

1.  Inhale in the Standing Foundation with your hands on your hips.

2.  Exhale and slide your right pointed foot forward. (Your toes stay in contact with the floor.)

3.  Inhale and point active toes.

4.  Exhale and draw a clockwise circle. Repeat four times.

5.  Inhale and point active toes.

6.  Exhale and draw a counterclockwise circle. Repeat four times.

7.  Inhale and return your right foot to the Standing Foundation. Shift to the left leg.

8.  Exhale and extend your right foot to the side. (Your toes stay in contact with the floor.)

9.  Inhale and point your toes.

10. Exhale and draw a clockwise circle. Repeat four times.

11. Inhale and point active toes.

12. Exhale and draw a counterclockwise circle. Repeat four times.

13. Inhale and return the right foot to active standing.

14. Repeat the sequence on the left leg.

# Level II

Adds a leg lift and active arms.

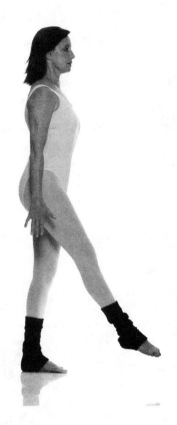

1. Inhale in the Standing Foundation with your arms at your sides and your fingers active.

2. Exhale and lift your right pointed foot three inches off the floor.

3. Inhale, toes active.

4. Exhale and draw small clockwise circles in the air. Repeat four times.

5. Inhale, toes active.

6. Exhale and reverse the direction of the circles. Repeat four times.

7. Inhale and exhale to return to the active Standing Foundation.

8. Repeat on the left leg.

# LEG CIRCLES
*(continued)*

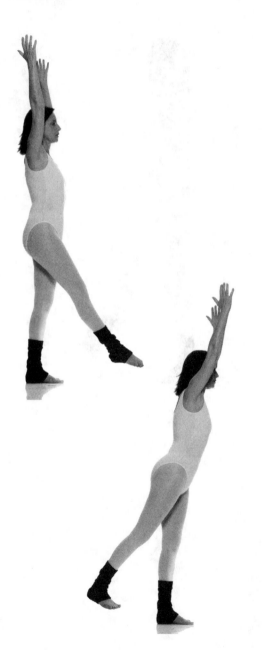

## Level III

Adds a higher leg lift, arm elevations, circles to the back, and continuous motion on one leg.

1. Inhale in the Standing Foundation with your arms at your sides.

2. Exhale, float your arms up to the ceiling, and lengthen your right pointed foot five inches off the floor.

3. Inhale and circle the leg five times clockwise.

4. Exhale and reverse the direction.

5. Inhale and move your right flexed foot to the side and do five clockwise circles.

6. Exhale and reverse the direction of the circles.

7. Inhale and hinge forward to move your right flexed foot back. Circle in one direction; then exhale and reverse the direction.

8. Inhale and return to the Standing Foundation with your arms by your sides.

9. Exhale to raise your arms to the ceiling and your center up.

10. Repeat on the left leg.

## Tall Technique

Imagine you have two sets of body headlights: the high beams at your hips and the low beams on the knees. The lights are beaming straight ahead during the entire exercise. Feel the quadricep muscles above the kneecaps pull up. Pay attention to the knees. If the beams point outward, turn the thigh bones inward without losing the foundation of the feet. If the beams go inward, rotate the thigh bones outward.

Maintain the lift of all the domes: the arch of the feet, the pelvic floor, the diaphragm, and the top of the head. Lengthening the spine can improve the alignment of the knees.

Activate your arms. Imagine light beams radiating out of each finger. To turn the finger beams on, your shoulder blades slide down your back and around your ribs below your armpits. The action of the shoulder blades will lengthen your arms. Inhale and then exhale to recharge your length.

## Goals

To stay active in your limbs while balancing. Good alignment engages your center and the lengthening of your entire spine. When lifting a leg in any direction, it should move without the pelvis unleveling. This will assist balance.

## Modifications

Make the circles smaller if your hips unlevel.

## Variations

Change speed. Do the front circles quickly, the ones to the side more slowly, and the ones to the back very slowly.

# 3 THE ROLL-UP
Pelvic Stability and Spinal Articulation

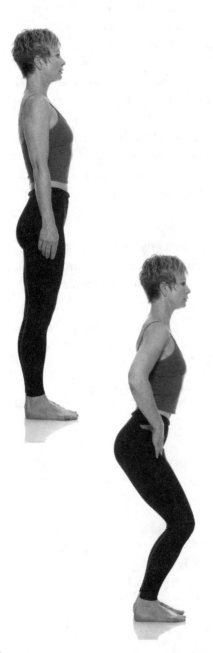

## Level I
Preparation

1. Inhale in the Standing Foundation with your hands by your sides.

2. Exhale to activate your legs, pressing both feet firmly into the floor.

3. Inhale and bend your knees.

4. Exhale, place your hands on your hips, and squat as if you are sitting on a chair.

5. Inhale and hold the position.

6. Exhale and contract the leg muscles to bring you to the Standing Foundation.

7. Repeat three more times.

# Level II

Adds spinal release and articulation.

1. Inhale in the standing foundation with your arms by your sides.

2. Exhale to activate your legs, pressing your feet firmly into the floor.

3. Inhale and bend the knees.

4. Exhale, bow forward, and release your spine over your legs so that your head and arms move toward the floor or as close as you can.

5. Inhale and feel the length of your body.

6. Exhale and contract your leg muscles to straighten the knees.

7. Inhale to roll up to the Standing Foundation.

8. Repeat the sequence four times.

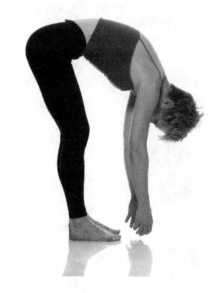

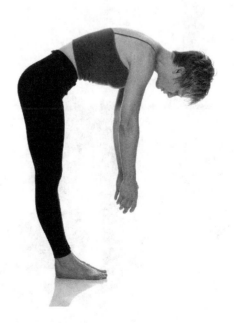

# THE ROLL-UP
*(continued)*

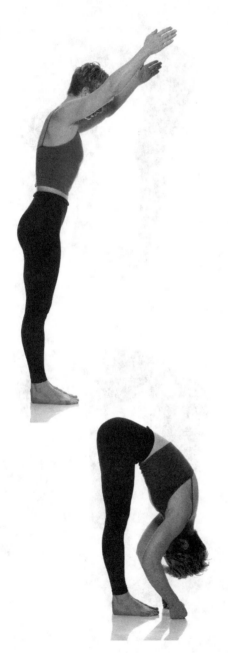

## Level III

Adds arm elevation.

1. Inhale in the Standing Foundation as you raise your arms high.

2. Exhale, bow, and roll down the spine as your arms follow the movement to as low as you can go.

3. Inhale and feel the length of the back body.

4. Exhale and press feet firmly down to activite legs.

5. Inhale to roll up.

6. Exhale to the Standing Foundation with arms at sides.

7. Repeat the sequence four times.

## Tall Technique

As you roll up, imagine your bones like individual dominoes building on top of each other; the shins over the ankles, the knees over the arches, the pelvis over the feet, the rib cage suspending over the pelvis, and the head floating above the rib cage. There is a plumb line that connects through the center of your head to your tailbone and heels in your standing posture.

Imagine your pelvic bones have feet. The sitting bones are the heels of each foot and the pubic bones are the toes. Place the pelvic feet over your real feet. Feel how the legs are working to maintain this position. Feel how organizing the pelvic "feet" over the standing feet deepens the connections.

## Goals

To use your legs dynamically. The legs initiate the movement of the spine. The legs work well when your pelvis is over your feet. The legs suspend the pelvis.

## Modifications

For tight hamstrings, bend your knees. For osteoporosis and disc injuries, practice only Level I with the squat.

## Variations

Roll up and down staying forward so that your leg muscles really work.

# 4 ROLLING LIKE A BALL

Full Spiral Flexion

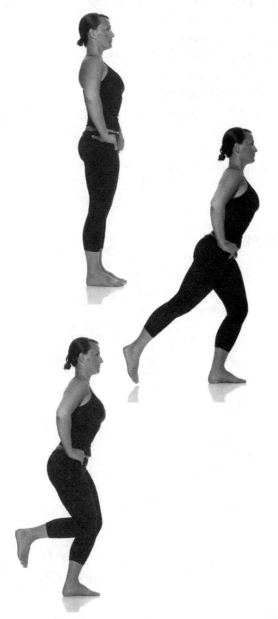

## Level I

Preparation

1. Inhale in the Standing Foundation with your hands on your hips.

2. Exhale and engage the pelvic floor.

3. Inhale and squat as if you are sitting on a chair with your hips and knees facing front.

4. Exhale while lifting your right foot up so your knee is in a 90-degree angle. You should look like a flamingo standing on one leg.

5. Inhale and extend your right leg back with your toes barely touching the floor.

6. Exhale and knee fold your right leg forward.

7. Inhale to hold the position.

8. Exhale to return the right foot to the Standing Foundation.

9. Repeat the sequence on left side.

10. Repeat two more sets.

## Level II

Adds single-leg balance and a full lunge.

1. Inhale in the Standing Foundation with your hands pressed together, fingers spread apart.

2. Exhale and bend your left knee while sliding your right leg straight back into a lunge. (The toes of the right foot are for balance. Your weight is on your left leg.)

3. Inhale and knee fold your right leg.

4. Exhale and bow over your hands.

5. Inhale and hold the position.

6. Exhale, unbow, and extend your right leg back.

7. Return to the Standing Foundation.

8. Repeat this entire sequence on the left leg. Make sure to inhale as you knee fold and exhale as you bow.

9. Inhale as you come to the Standing Foundation.

10. Repeat the sequence twice on each side.

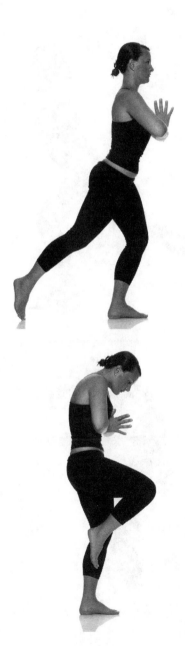

# ROLLING LIKE A BALL
*(continued)*

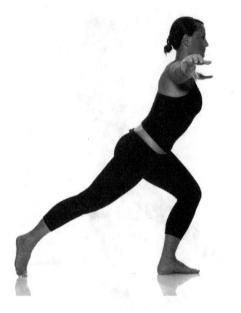

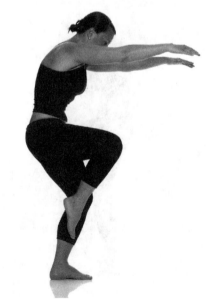

### Level III

Adds the movement of the arms to the sides and front.

1. Inhale in the Standing Foundation and raise your arms to the sides at shoulder height.

2. Exhale, bend the left knee, and slide the right leg back into a lunge.

3. Inhale and shift your weight onto your left bent leg.

4. Exhale, knee fold the right leg forward, bow, and reach your arms forward.

5. Inhale to hold the position.

6. Repeat the entire sequence. Remember to exhale as you bow and inhale to unbow and knee fold.

7. Repeat three sets for each leg.

8. To end, press the feet down to lift the torso up to your best Standing Foundation.

## Tall Technique

Imagine that from your sitting bones there are Greek columns rising within your torso. These columns lift your rib cage equally up and away from your pelvis, front, back, and sides. Your shoulder girdle is riding on top of your rib cage and the columns. If you collapse the rib cage during movement, balance and control will be compromised.

Maintain the lift of your torso as you keep your knee over your foot. Your knee stays bent and remains over the ankle in line with the second and third toes of your other foot.

When you extend your leg backward, imagine that it is on a track. Your bent knee and ankle are aligned over a parallel track. Feel your extended lunge leg reaching in the opposite direction of your bent leg.

With your arms reaching forward, deepen the curve of the spine by reaching your waist backward. You are creating a countertension of the arms as you reach forward while your waist is curving backward.

## Goals

To learn complex choreography that forces your brain to work. Awareness of your body reaching in opposite directions centers your core.

## Modifications

If needed, touch a wall to maintain balance.

## Variations

Change the rhythm and speed. Deepen the lunge.

# 5 SINGLE-LEG STRETCH
Trunk Stability with Forward Flexion and Hip Differentiation

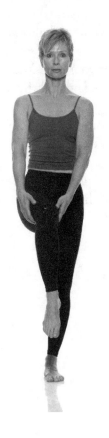

## Level 1
Preparation

1. Inhale in the Standing Foundation with your arms at your sides.

2. Exhale, knee fold your right leg, placing your hands under your thigh to support it.

3. Inhale and exhale two breath cycles while holding your knee.

4. Inhale to return the leg to the floor to the Standing Foundation.

5. Repeat with the left leg.

6. Repeat the sequence twice for each leg.

# Level II

Adds the Bow and hands at the knee.

1. Inhale in the Standing Foundation with your arms by your sides.

2. Exhale, bow, and knee fold your right knee, placing both hands around the front of the knee for support.

3. Inhale and exhale two breath cycles while holding the position.

4. Inhale, release the knee, and straighten your spine to return to the Standing Foundation.

5. Repeat the entire movement for the left side.

6. Repeat the entire sequence six times, alternating legs.

7. Inhale and return to the Standing Foundation.

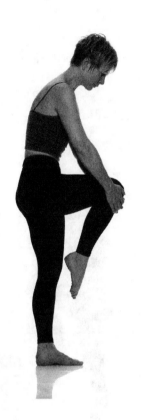

# SINGLE-LEG STRETCH

*(continued)*

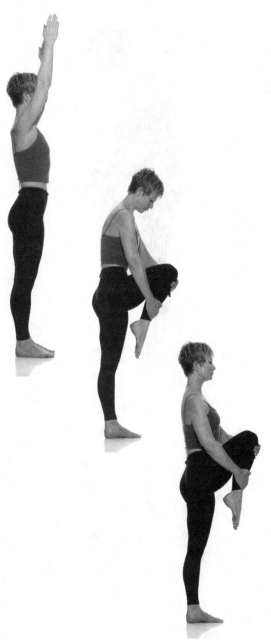

## Level III

Adds arm-level changes and a more complex hand placement.

1. Inhale and stand with your arms raised to the ceiling.

2. Exhale while bowing and knee folding the right leg. Grasp your knee with your left hand and your ankle with your right hand.

3. Inhale and straighten your spine while deepening the Knee Fold.

4. Exhale and release the right knee to the Standing Foundation.

5. Repeat three times and shift to the left leg for four repetitions.

6. Repeat the sequence twice.

## Tall Technique

Look in the mirror and organize the alignment of your feet, knees, pelvis, and rib cage over each other. Your spine extends to the roof of your mouth. Feel your mouth dome float up.

Check in the mirror that your hips are level. This is necessary to maintain balance when you knee fold.

Remember the Bow comes from the upper spine only. The lower ribs should remain centered over the pelvis.

## Goals

To knee fold with hips level. The ribs lengthen away from the pelvis as you ground the legs and feet.

## Modifications

Touch a wall for balance.

## Variations

Close your eyes during this exercise. This reduces proprioception—your sense of where your body is in space—by 30 percent!

# 6 DOUBLE-LEG STRETCH

Pelvic Stability and Full Breathing

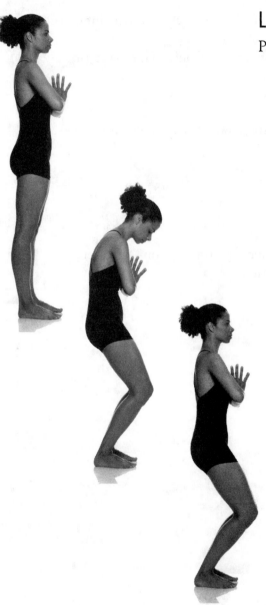

## Level I

Preparation

1. Inhale in the Standing Foundation with hands in prayer position.

2. Exhale, bow, and knee bend.

3. Inhale to straighten your spine.

4. Exhale and straighten your legs to return to active Standing Foundation.

5. Repeat twice more, using each breath to open the ribs front and back.

6. To end, return to the Standing Foundation and repeat two breath cycles to feel full rib cage expansion.

## Level II

Adds hands behind the knees.

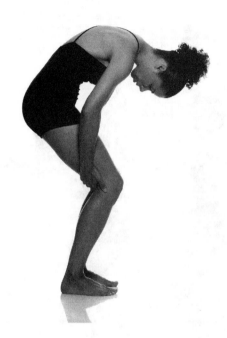

1. Inhale in the Standing Foundation with arms by your sides.
2. Exhale, knee bend, and bow, bringing your hands to your knees.
3. Inhale to widen the back ribs and place your hands behind your knees with the elbows out to the side.
4. Exhale to engage the abdominals to stretch the upper back ribs toward the ceiling.
5. Inhale to release your hands.
6. Exhale and straighten your legs.
7. Inhale and roll up to standing.
8. Repeat three times.

# DOUBLE-LEG STRETCH
*(continued)*

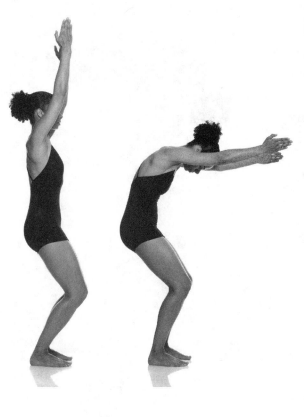

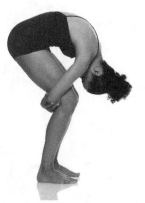

## Level III

Adds arm-level shifts and more resistance.

1. Inhale in the Standing Foundation.

2. Exhale and float your arms up toward the ceiling as you knee bend.

3. Inhale and hold the position.

4. Exhale and bow. Your arms move forward with the torso.

5. Inhale and drop your arms behind your knees, bringing the opposite hand to the opposite elbow.

6. Exhale to lift the abdominals up, stretching your upper back toward the ceiling. Release the head.

7. Inhale to release your arms.

8. Exhale to activate the legs, pressing your feet into the floor.

9. Inhale to roll up to the Standing Foundation.

8. Repeat three more times.

## Tall Technique

The benefits from full breathing are numerous. The breath can open space between the ribs. The prayer hands will help soften your breastbone into your back ribs.

Keep shoulders, hips, and knees facing front. When you are stretching your upper back, a countertension develops between your shoulder blades, reaching to the ceiling as your arms stretch.

Tightness in the upper body restricts breathing and prevents the torso from lengthening. Practice deepening each inhalation and exhalation so that your breath will assist you.

## Goals

To attain fluidity of movement in several positions.

## Modifications

If flexing of the upper spine is contraindicated, eliminate the Bow. Instead wrap your arms around your chest to reach your shoulder blades. Inhale to help open the tightness between the shoulder blades.

## Variations

Roll up to standing and then up to releve. Hold for one breath cycle and then slowly release your heels to the floor.

# 7 SPINE STRETCH
Spinal Articulation from the Lumbar

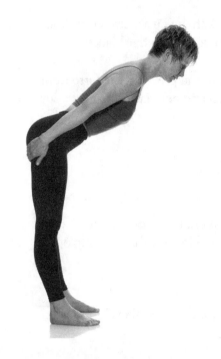

## Level I
Preparation

1. Inhale to stand with your feet parallel, wider than hip distance apart, and hands at the gluteal fold (under the buttocks).

2. Exhale and hinge forward 45 degrees at the hip with a neutral spine.

3. Inhale to hold the position without letting your legs move backward.

4. Exhale to press the feet into the floor and deepen the hinge to a 90-degree angle.

5. Inhale to bring yourself back to the Standing Foundation.

6. Repeat four times.

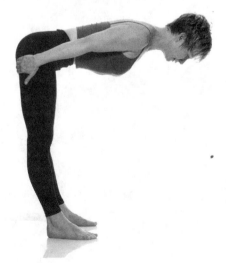

# Level II

Adds arms wide and flexion of the coccyx/lumbar.

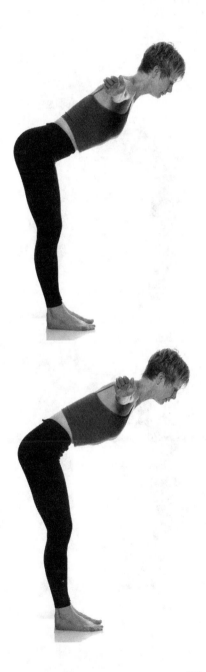

1. Inhale with your legs wide and raise your arms from your back out to the sides at shoulder height.

2. Exhale and hinge forward at your hips with a neutral spine.

3. Inhale and lengthen your spine away from your active legs.

4. Exhale to curl your tail (coccyx) under.

5. Inhale and lengthen back to a neutral spine in the hinge position.

6. Exhale to activate your legs.

7. Inhale to return to standing.

8. Repeat four times.

# SPINE STRETCH
*(continued)*

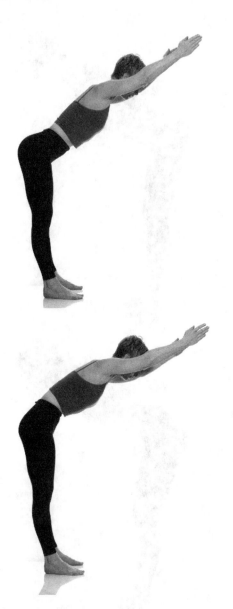

## Level III

Adds arms high to increase the lever of the top body.

1. Inhale as you lift your arms up to the ceiling, palms facing each other, with your legs wide.

2. Exhale to hinge at your hips with a neutral spine (your arms stay in line with your ears).

3. Inhale and keep lengthening your spine away from your active legs.

4. Exhale and curl the tailbone under, using your abdominals only. In this position your legs are not working as actively.

5. Inhale and lengthen back to a neutral spine parallel to the floor (or to your own ability).

6. Exhale to reactivate your legs into greater length.

7. Inhale to return to standing with your arms reaching over your head to ceiling.

8. Repeat four times.

## Tall Technique

Bring awareness to your sitting bones. Imagine the bones are moving closer to the pubic bones. During exhalation, dome up the pelvic floor. Feel how this strengthens your legs.

Your spine is moving forward as your pelvis pivots on top of your thigh bones. Move the spine in one piece forward and back by using your leg and hip muscles with a lengthened spine.

Curling the coccyx (tailbone) is initiated with your abdominals only. Extending the arms out in front increases the lever of the torso.

## Goals

To return to standing using your legs. Imagine you are a dunking bird that goes up and down to drink water from a bowl.

The connection of your legs into your pelvis brings the pelvis up, forward, and back. Imagine your pelvis is riding high on top of your thigh bones.

## Modifications

If you lack the flexibility and/or strength to extend your spine to the tabletop position, go to the position where you can maintain a neutral spine.

## Variations

Do not allow the legs to move backward when you hinge your spine forward.

# 8 OPEN-LEG ROCKER

Promotes Stability in Motion

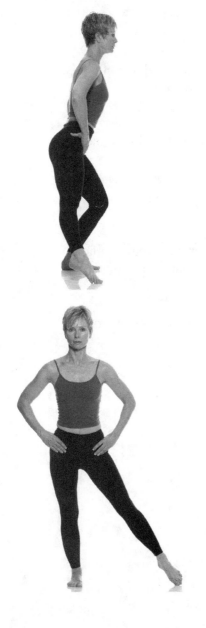

## Level I

Preparation

1. Inhale while standing with your legs in a wide parallel position with hands on your hips.

2. Exhale to lift your abdominals up as you bend your knees.

3. Inhale and shift your weight to your right leg in a modified side lunge. (Think of yourself as a speed skater with your torso staying in neutral.)

4. Exhale to straighten your right leg. The toe of your left foot will stay in contact with the floor.

5. Inhale to bend your right knee and shift your weight back to center. Both knees are bent.

6. Exhale to straighten both legs.

7. Inhale in the Standing Foundation with legs in a wide parallel.

8. Exhale to bend both legs.

9. Inhale and shift your weight to your left leg in a modified side lunge.

10. Exhale to straighten your left leg. Your right toe stays in contact with the floor.

11. Inhale to shift your weight back to center.

12. Exhale to straighten both legs.

13. Repeat the entire set two times.

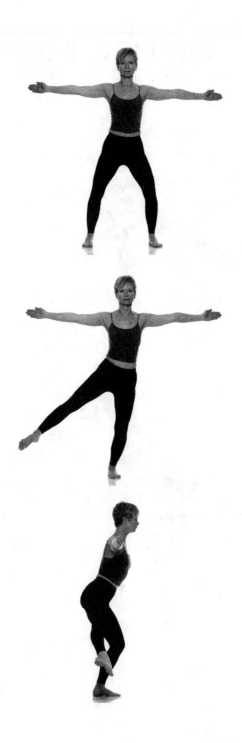

## Level II

Adds arms out to the sides, which widens the body so that it works harder.

1. Inhale, standing with legs wide, arms reaching out to the sides.
2. Exhale as you bend your knees.
3. Inhale and shift your weight to your right leg in a side lunge.
4. Exhale to straighten your right leg. The toe of your left foot will come slightly off the floor.
5. Inhale to bend your right knee and shift your weight back to center.
6. Exhale to bend knees.
7. Inhale to shift your weight to your left leg.
8. Exhale to straighten your left leg. The toe of your right foot will come slightly off the floor.
9. Inhale and shift your weight to center.
10. Exhale to straighten both legs and return to active standing.
11. Repeat the entire set three times.

# OPEN-LEG ROCKER
*(continued)*

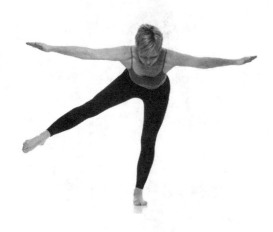

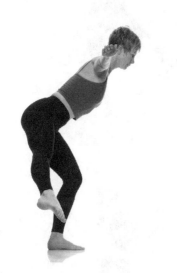

## Level III

Adds the hinge, which forces your legs to work harder.

1. Inhale while standing with your legs in a wide parallel, arms reaching out to the sides.
2. Exhale, squat, and hinge the spine forward from the hip, parallel to the floor.
3. Inhale and transfer your body weight over your right leg with the spine leaning forward.
4. Exhale in the hinge position and straighten the right leg; the left leg will lift off the floor a few inches.
5. Inhale and bend the right leg again.
6. Exhale to return to the squatting position with the spine forward.
7. Inhale and transfer your body weight over your left leg with the spine leaning forward.
8. Exhale in the hinge position and straighten the left leg, which naturally lifts the right foot off the floor.
9. Inhale and bend the left leg again.
10. Exhale and return to the squatting position with the spine forward.
11. Inhale and engage the thigh and hip muscles to bring the spine back to an erect standing position.
12. Repeat the entire sequence four times.

## Tall Technique

Lateral shifting requires good ankle and knee alignment. Pay attention to pulling up the kneecap to activate the thigh muscles to straighten the leg. The other foot will lift off the floor as you contract the muscles of the active leg. One foot leaves the floor because the opposite knee is straightening. Feel how the arm connection to the back helps to lift the foot higher off the floor.

Active arms help lift the ribs up. Reaching the elbows away from the tips of the shoulder blades gives the back support.

## Goals

To correct lateral shifting essential for the health of the knees. Bending and straightening the knee is the action of walking up the stairs. When you align the knees, the upper body is lifted and lighter.

## Modifications

Practice lateral shifts to a modified side lunge.

## Variations

Hinge your spine forward to 90 degrees if you can maintain the neutral position. Increase the speed of the lateral shifts.

# 9  SPINE TWIST
Spinal Rotation and One-Leg Balance

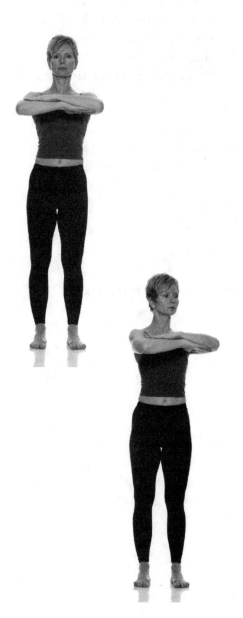

## Level I

Preparation

1. Inhale in the Standing Foundation with your arms crossed in front of your chest like a genie.

2. Exhale and firmly press your feet into the floor to activate the legs.

3. Inhale while floating your ribs away from your pelvis and twist to your right side (your nose stays in line with the breast bone).

4. Exhale to lift and rotate your upper torso back to the center.

5. Inhale to spiral your ribs to the left side.

6. Exhale to return to the center.

7. Repeat for three sets.

# Level II

Adds instability and increases the spiral mass with the arms extended.

1. Inhale and stand with parallel legs that are close together so that the feet touch.

2. Exhale and reach your arms out to the sides at shoulder height.

3. Inhale and twist your spine to the right.

4. Exhale to return to the center.

5. Inhale and spiral to the left.

6. Exhale to return to the center.

7. Repeat for four sets.

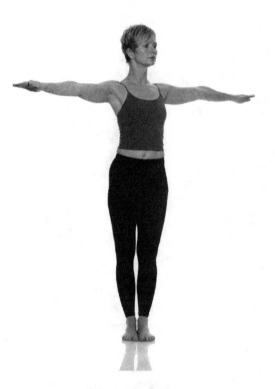

# SPINE TWIST
*(continued)*

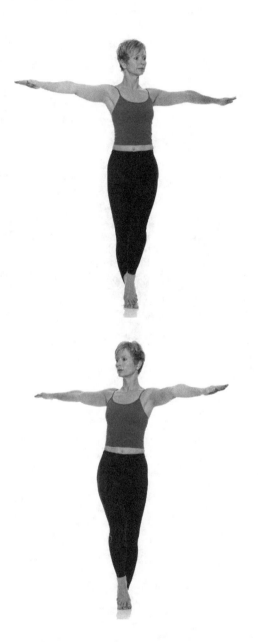

## Level III

Really reduces the foot stability platform since you are now on one leg.

1. Inhale and stand on your right leg only with your arms out to the sides at shoulder height.
2. Exhale and put your left foot on your right foot.
3. Inhale and twist to the right.
4. Exhale and spiral back to the center.
5. Inhale and twist to the left.
6. Exhale, spiral back to the center, and stand on both feet.
7. Inhale to shift to the left leg.
8. Exhale and put the right foot on top of the left one.
9. Inhale and twist to the right.
10. Exhale and spiral back to the center.
11. Inhale and twist to the left.
12. Exhale, spiral back to the center, and stand on both feet.
13. Repeat each left/right set four times.

## Tall Technique

Imagine there are teacups on each of your shoulders and elbows. You must keep the teacups level with rotation. Your elbows stay in line with your shoulders throughout the twist. This is a spinal movement of your torso, not your shoulders. Imagine you have headlights on your hips and on your knees. They need to be focused forward throughout the rotation. When you rotate, maintain equal space around the spine from the ribs to the hips. The nose stays in line with the breastbone. The head moves only because the ribs move. Keep the teacups quiet and the headlights focused forward.

With each exhalation, lift the domes of your pelvic floor, rib cage, and mouth higher. Imagine that the space from your ribs to your hips is covered with a wet towel. As you twist, you are trying to wring the water out of the towel.

When your arms are wide to the sides at shoulder height, imagine you are wearing a yoke: a bar over your shoulders with two pails hanging from ropes at the end of the bar. When you twist, the pails stay level. The bar is your shoulder girdle and arms. This bar does not change position on the back of your shoulders as you move.

## Goals

To learn to stabilize the lower body as you twist the upper body with length is essential. Think of your torso as a Slinky toy. This toy is a series of spirals that become longer when pulled apart.

## Modifications

Perform Level I with your hands on your waist and your elbows pointing out to the sides.

## Variations

Rotate your head in the opposite direction of your spiraled torso.

# 10 THE CORKSCREW

Pelvic Rotation and Complex Choreography

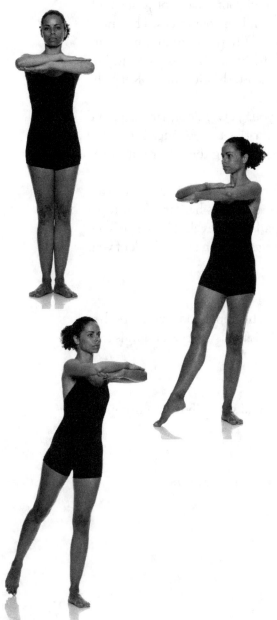

## Level I

Preparation

1. Inhale and stand with your legs in first position.

2. Exhale and cross your arms one on top of the other with elbows aligned to your shoulders.

3. Inhale to rotate your upper body to the right as your right foot reaches to the front right corner.

4. Exhale to rotate your upper body to the left as you circle your right leg to the back right corner.

5. Inhale to return to the starting position.

6. Repeat two more sets for this side.

7. Inhale to rotate your upper body to the left as your left foot reaches to the front left corner.

8. Exhale to rotate your upper body to the right as you circle your left leg to the back left corner.

9. Inhale to return to the starting position.

10. Repeat the sequence two more sets for this side.

## Level II

Adds longer arms (more to spiral) and one-leg balance.

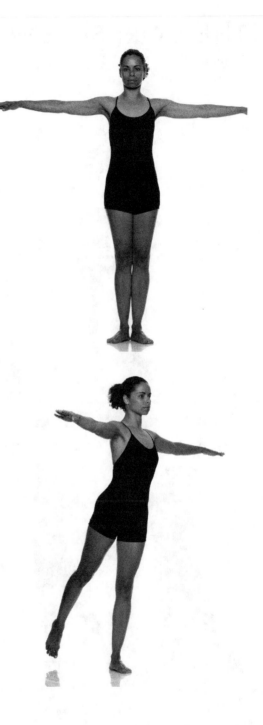

1. Inhale and stand with your legs in first position.

2. Exhale and float your arms out to the sides at shoulder level.

3. Inhale to rotate your upper body to the right as your right foot reaches to the front right corner and is lifted two inches off the floor.

4. Exhale to rotate your upper body to the left as you circle your right lifted leg to the back right corner.

5. Inhale to return to the starting position.

6. Repeat two more sets for this side.

7. Exhale and float arms out to sides at shoulder level.

8. Inhale to rotate your upper body to the left as your left foot reaches to the front left corner and is lifted two inches off the floor.

9. Exhale to rotate your upper body to the right as you circle your left lifted leg to the back left corner.

10. Inhale to return to the starting position.

11. Repeat the sequence two more sets for this side.

# THE CORKSCREW
*(continued)*

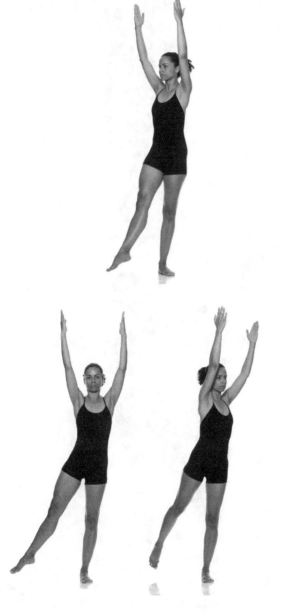

## Level III

Adds arms in a high V position.

1. Inhale and stand with your legs in first position.

2. Exhale and raise your arms to the ceiling in the shape of the letter V.

3. Inhale with your arms lifted. Twist your upper spine to your right as your lifted right leg reaches to the right front corner of the room.

4. Exhale as you circle the lifted right leg to the right side; the torso twists center.

5. Inhale with the arms lifted, the spine twisting left as the right foot circles to the back right diagonal. Your right leg stays lifted the entire time.

6. Repeat two more sets.

7. Exhale and return to the starting position.

8. Repeat with the left leg.

9. Repeat two more sets.

## Tall Technique

Imagine your spine is three spheres: the pelvis, the rib cage, and the head float above each other. The spheres are different sizes, but there is a plumb line connecting them.

When your arms reach to the sides at shoulder level, the shoulder blades imprint toward the side ribs. Scapula stability increases spinal rotation and lifts the rib cage sphere.

Coordination of the arms and the leg circling comes from the spinal rotation. Imagine your upper body like the lazy Susan at the dinner table. It is suspended above your standing legs.

## Goals

To coordinate complex movements with rotation. When the torso and hips twist in opposite directions, focus on the fluidity and length of the movement.

## Modifications

Put your hands on your waist with the elbows facing out for greater stability. Separate the lower body movement from the upper body motion.

## Variations

Releve when your arms are up and your leg circles to the side. Return from releve when twisting to the diagonals.

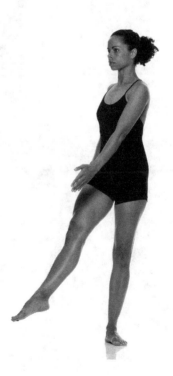

# 11 THE SAW

Spinal Rotation and Hip Differentiation

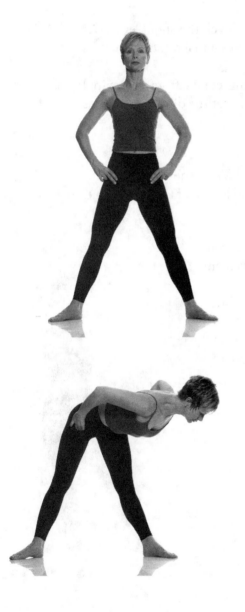

## Level I

Preparation

1. Inhale to stand with your legs wide in the turn-out position with your hands on the front of your hips.

2. Exhale to activate your feet and hands to lengthen your torso away from your lower body.

3. Inhale and twist your lengthened torso to the right, facing the front diagonal.

4. Exhale as you hinge forward at the hips over your right leg, bringing a neutral torso parallel to the floor (if possible).

5. Inhale and activate the back leg muscles to bring your torso back to standing.

6. Exhale and twist your torso to the front, returning to center.

7. Inhale and twist your lengthened torso to the left, facing the front diagonal.

8. Exhale and lengthen your spine as you fold at the hips over your left leg.

9. Inhale, engage the legs, and return to standing.

10. Exhale and twist your torso to the front, returning to center.

11. Repeat two sets.

# Level II

Adds arm choreography, with rotation.

1. Inhale to stand with your legs wide in the turn-out position.

2. Exhale to raise your arms to the ceiling in the letter V.

3. Inhale to twist to your right side.

4. Exhale as you hinge at your hips forward over your right leg.

5. Inhale and hold the position.

6. Exhale to release your spine and arms over your right leg.

7. Inhale to straighten the spine to the hinge position.

8. Exhale, lengthen the spine, and activate the legs.

9. Inhale and return to standing, still facing the front right diagonal.

10. Exhale and twist your spine to the center.

11. Repeat the entire sequence on the left side.

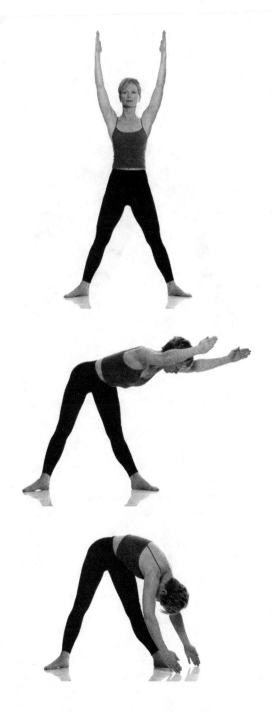

# THE SAW

*(continued)*

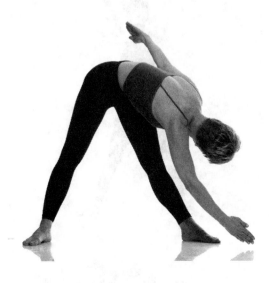

## Level III

Adds pulses ("saw") and arm variation.

1. Inhale to stand with your legs wide in the turn-out position.

2. Exhale to raise your arms to the ceiling in the letter V.

3. Inhale and twist to your right side.

4. Exhale as you hinge at your hips forward over your right leg.

5. Inhale and hold the position.

6. Exhale to release your spine over your right leg. The left arm reaches to the right toes as the right arm reaches back.

7. Inhale to straighten the spine to the hinge position. Arms reach in a wide V.

8. Exhale, lengthen the spine, and activate your legs.

9. Inhale. Return to standing, still facing the right diagonal with your arms reaching up to the ceiling in a wide V.

10. Exhale and twist your spine to the center.

11. Repeat the entire sequence on the left side.

## Tall Technique

Rotation is usually easier on one side. In the hinge position, maintain a neutral torso parallel to the floor if possible. Watch that your knees don't shift or lock when you "saw."

Increase the lengthening of your spine before you fold at the hips. Don't allow your legs to move back. If you let go of your legs, the sequencing of the movement is not as fluid.

## Goals

Activation of your legs allows your spine more freedom to rotate, which will narrow your waist. Paying attention to your working legs yields new spaces between your vertebrae to twist and release.

## Modifications

Bend your knees if short hamstrings restrict movement.

## Variations

Close your eyes for one repetition.

# 12 ROLL-DOWN TO SWAN
Level Changes, Spinal Extension, and Several Positions

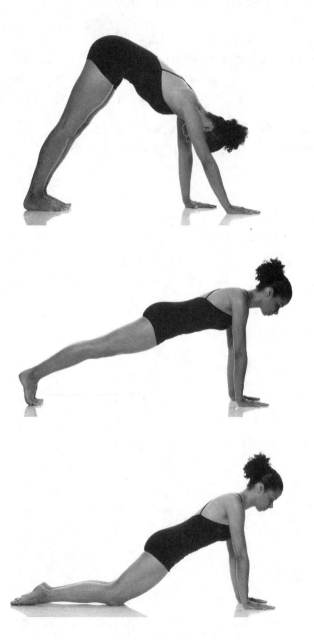

## Level I
Modified plank

1. Inhale in the Standing Foundation with your arms by your sides.

2. Exhale, bow, and roll down, bringing your hands to the floor.

3. Inhale and walk your hands out away from your feet into a plank position.

4. Exhale and lower your knees to the floor.

5. Inhale and exhale and hold this position for three breath cycles.

6. Inhale to return to the plank position.

7. Exhale and walk your hands back toward your feet.

8. Inhale and roll up to the Standing Foundation.

9. Repeat three sets.

# Level II

Adds a sequence of upper body extension (modified swan).

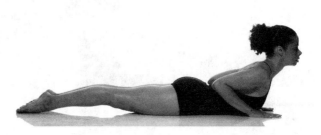

1. Inhale in the Standing Foundation with your arms by your sides.

2. Exhale to bow and roll down, bringing your hands to the floor.

3. Inhale as you walk your hands out to the plank position.

4. Exhale to bring your knees to the floor and bend your elbows close to your sides. Your front body lowers to the floor.

5. Inhale, press the front of your thighs into the floor, and extend the spine and straighten the arms to the modified swan.

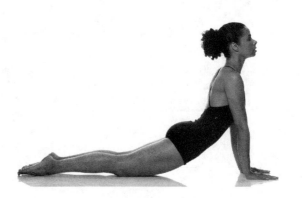

6. Exhale as you reach your heels backward to extend the legs to plank position.

7. Inhale to hold the plank.

8. Exhale and walk the hands back toward the feet. The torso is hanging forward.

9. Inhale to roll up to the Standing Foundation.

10. Repeat five sets.

# ROLL-DOWN TO SWAN
*(continued)*

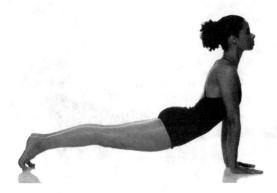

## Level III

Adds the full swan, which requires you to distribute your weight along your body.

1. Inhale in the Standing Foundation.

2. Exhale to bow and roll down, bringing your hands to the floor.

3. Inhale as you walk your hands out to the plank position.

4. Exhale to hold the position.

5. Inhale to move to the swan by activating your legs backward as your spine extends forward in opposition.

6. Exhale to deepen the connections of your legs, arms, and torso in this extension.

7. Inhale and go to the plank position.

8. Exhale and walk your hands back to the feet and hold for three breath cycles.

9. Repeat the plank to swan four times.

10. Inhale and return to the Standing Foundation.

## Tall Technique

Keep the legs active. Do not allow the legs to move backward as you roll down. Lifting the pelvic dome helps distribute your weight.

Position your hands directly under your shoulders with fingers spread wide. Imagine lifting your torso from the floor with your arm bones.

In the pike, imagine a harness around the front of your hips lifting the lower abs and pelvic dome. This will suspend your hips while your heels lower toward the floor. Connecting the arms into your shoulder blades will make this position easier.

In the plank position, pay attention to active feet and hands. Maintain a long, unbroken line from the front of your lower ribs, hips, and knees. If you feel the movement in your back, you are not giving enough muscular support on all sides of the body. Connect your hands and feet into the floor to support your torso.

## Goals

To be weight-bearing on your arms and legs simultaneously. The opposition of reaching your feet and hands into the floor will power your middle to new strength.

## Modifications

If your hamstrings are tight, bend your knees and hinge the front of your hips on your thighs. Stand with your heels against a wall. The wall will buttress and add support.

## Variations

Do the exercise with two full breaths on each pose.

# 13 LEG KICK-BACK

Single-Leg Balance and Spinal Extension

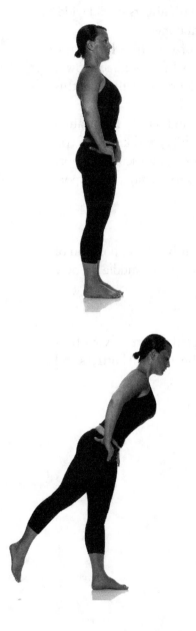

## Level I

Preparation

1. Inhale in the Standing Foundation.

2. Exhale and activate your legs and place your hands on your hip bones.

3. Inhale and slide your right leg backward as if it were on a track.

4. Exhale and hinge slightly forward. The right toes lift slightly off the floor during the hinge (seesaw).

5. Inhale as the head moves toward the floor and the back of your right leg lifts toward the ceiling. The body and right leg are parallel to the floor.

6. Exhale and activate your left standing leg. Your spine remains long with your head and tail in line.

7. Inhale. Unhinge and bring the spine straight up while simultaneously returning the right foot to the floor.

8. Repeat three seesaws on your right side; this action causes your body to pivot forward and backward on your stabilized leg.

9. Inhale and return to the Standing Foundation. Do four seesaws on your other side.

# Level II

Adds a knee bend and greater range of spine extension.

1. Inhale in the Standing Foundation with your arms at shoulder height.

2. Exhale to reach your arms behind you so that you can interlace your fingers and lengthen them toward the floor.

3. Inhale to extend the upper back and lift the breastbone to the ceiling as the head follows.

4. Exhale to bring the spine into neutral and slide your right foot backward.

5. Inhale to open the arms to the sides.

6. Exhale to hinge forward (seesaw).

7. Inhale to bend the right knee.

8. Exhale to straighten the right knee, keeping a long line from head to toe.

9. Inhale and return to the Standing Foundation.

10. Repeat on the left side.

11. Perform the series three times.

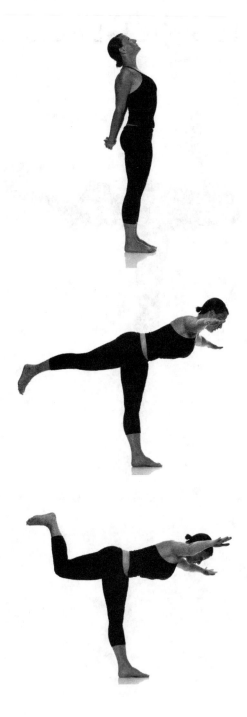

# LEG KICK-BACK

*(continued)*

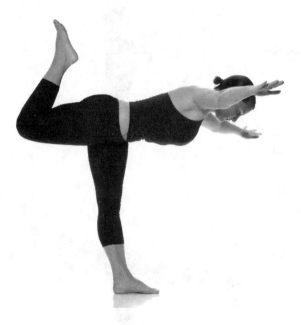

## Level III

Adds quick, sharp kicks.

1. Inhale in the Standing Foundation with your arms at shoulder height.

2. Exhale to reach your arms behind you so that you can interlace your fingers and lengthen them toward the floor.

3. Inhale to extend the upper back and lift your breastbone to the ceiling as the head follows.

4. Exhale to bring the spine into neutral and slide your right foot backward.

5. Inhale and open your arms to the sides.

6. Exhale and hinge forward (seesaw).

7. Inhale to kick the right foot toward your buttocks in a sharp movement.

8. Exhale to release the right foot straight backward. Repeat three times.

9. Inhale, keeping a long line from head to toe. Return to the Standing Foundation.

10. Repeat on the left side.

11. Perform the series three times.

## Tall Technique

Imagine your body as a seesaw as you hinge with a long line from head to tail. The sitting bones do not change as you perform this exercise. Correct position forces your standing leg to work.

Feel how the upper back spine extension opens the chest. In the seesaw position, the standing leg must stay strongly aligned with the knee over the ankle. Work your standing foot for better stability. Keep the head aligned with your lifted leg as you rock on top of your standing leg. Connect all of your body parts to balance.

## Goals

To gain length and fluidity of the moving body on the standing leg. As your strength and flexibility increase, your body will resist gravity in standing.

To maintain alignment of the standing leg so that your outside thigh muscles work.

## Modifications

Touch—don't hold—a chair back for balance.

## Variations

Alternate pointing and flexing the foot that does the kicking.

# 14 NECK PULL

Spinal Sequencing and One-Leg Balance

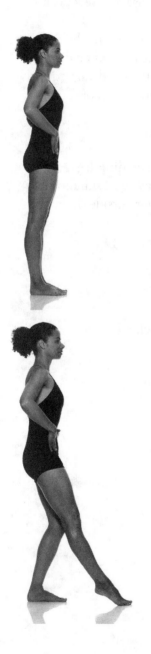

## Level I

Preparation

1. Inhale in the Standing Foundation with your hands on your hips.

2. Exhale to engage your pelvic floor.

3. Inhale to slide your right foot out to the front.

4. Exhale to plié (bend) your standing left leg.

5. Inhale and imagine reaching the right foot out farther.

6. Exhale to straighten the left leg and simultaneously slide the right leg back to the Standing Foundation position.

7. Inhale and slide your left foot forward.

8. Exhale and plié the right standing leg.

9. Inhale to reach the left leg out farther.

10. Exhale to straighten the right leg and slide the left leg back to the Standing Foundation.

11. Repeat three times.

# Level II

Adds the Bow, the prayer hands, and a leg lift.

1. Inhale in the Standing Foundation.

2. Exhale to move your hands into your breastbone in prayer position.

3. Inhale to slide the right leg forward.

4. Exhale, bow, and simultaneously plié the left leg.

5. Inhale and lift the right leg off the floor several inches or to your own ability.

6. Exhale and lower the right foot to the floor.

7. Inhale to straighten your spine as you unplié your left leg and slide your right leg back, returning to the Standing Foundation.

8. Repeat the sequence on the left side.

9. Repeat the entire sequence four times.

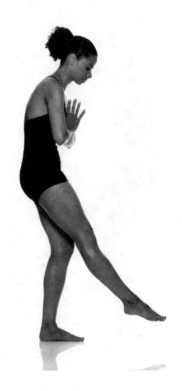

# NECK PULL
*(continued)*

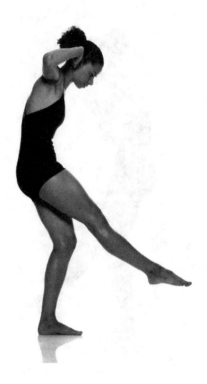

## Level III

Adds the challenge of holding the arms up as you simultaneously flex and balance on one leg.

1. Inhale in the Standing Foundation with your hands laced behind your head and your elbows reaching to the sides.

2. Exhale, bow, and plié.

3. Inhale and lift your right leg.

4. Exhale to deepen the Bow and the leg lift.

5. Inhale to simultaneously straighten your spine, then lower the right leg and unplié the left leg and return to active standing.

6. Repeat the complete sequence three times on one leg, then switch to the other leg.

7. Repeat the sequence, but alternate legs for four more sets as in Level II.

## Tall Technique

Check the position of your pelvis in the mirror. The pelvic triangle has three points in front: two hip bones and the pubis. Maintain the pelvic triangle's symmetry. Plié and straighten your legs without changing the plane of the pelvic triangle. Do not tuck, because this will bring the pubic bone in front of the hip bones. Stay connected.

On the foot of your standing leg, feel the four corners and the edges on the floor.

In the Bow position, move the hands into your breastbone and feel your front ribs soften into the back body. Feel the width of your back ribs without losing the natural curve of your waist. You should feel as if you are sitting on a chair.

Imagine a puppet string attached to your back, which will suspend your rib cage up to the ceiling throughout the movement. If you crunch rather than bow, you will lose balance.

## Goals

To stay long and even as you bend your body in two places.

## Modifications

Touch a wall for balance.

## Variations

Extend your upper spine to swan and alternate between this and the Bow position.

# 15 SIDE KICK

Differentiation of the Hip with Leg Mobility

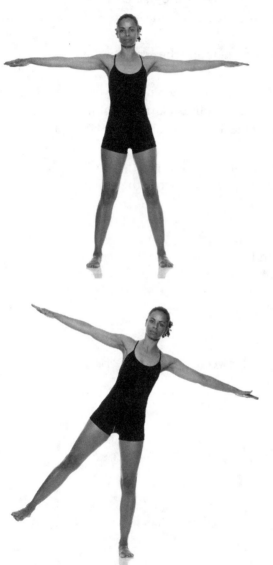

## Level I

Preparation

1.  Inhale and stand with your arms reaching out at shoulder height and your legs wider than hip distance in parallel.
2.  Exhale and feel your entire body lengthened in space.
3.  Inhale and slide your right flexed foot out to the side as far as possible.
4.  Exhale to side bend to the left at your hip, which should lift your right leg three inches. Hold this position for a complete inhalation and exhalation.
5.  Inhale to return to the center, lowering your foot.
6.  Exhale to stand with the legs wider than the hips, feet pressing down, and arms out to your sides.
7.  Inhale to slide your left flexed foot to the side.
8.  Exhale and tilt your spine to the right, which lifts your left foot. Hold for a full inhalation and exhalation.
9.  Inhale to return to the center, lowering your foot.
10. Repeat three sets.

## Level II

Adds a pivot.

1. Inhale to stand with your arms out to your sides at shoulder height.

2. Exhale to energize your total body.

3. Inhale and tilt your spine to the left so that your right flexed foot lifts off the floor about three inches.

4. Exhale to pivot your torso to the diagonal. Hold for a full inhalation and exhalation.

5. Inhale to return to the center.

6. Exhale and lower your leg to stand with your legs wider than your hips.

7. Repeat with the left leg.

8. Repeat three more sets.

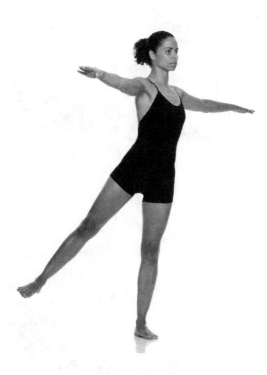

# SIDE KICK
*(continued)*

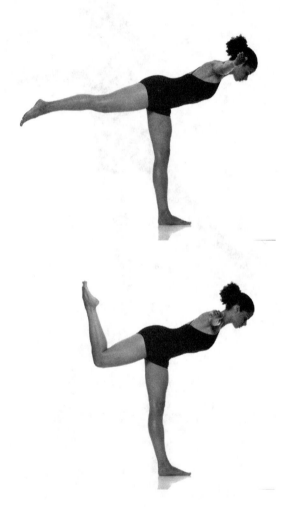

## Level III

Adds a high leg lift and a bigger seesaw and kicks.

1. Inhale to stand with your arms out to the sides at shoulder height.
2. Exhale to lift up your arches and head.
3. Inhale to tilt to the left, lifting the right flexed foot about five inches.
4. Exhale to pivot your body on your left standing leg. Seesaw the spine lower as the right leg moves higher.
5. Inhale and bend the right knee.
6. Exhale and straighten the right knee.
7. Inhale to pivot back to the side tilt with the right foot five inches off the floor.
8. Exhale to standing with legs slightly wider than the hips.
9. Repeat with the left leg.
10. Return to standing with parallel legs wider than hips.
11. Repeat for four sets.

## Tall Technique

For greater awareness of the side dimensions, reach your fingertips to touch the sides of the room. Radiate the sides of your entire body to the left and right walls. Imagine that there are multiple puppet strings gently pulling you in various directions and planes to give you balance and support.

Energize your total body while feeling the opposition from your head reaching up and your tail reaching down, the left side away from your right side, and focus on the facings of your front and back body. Face your hips, knees, and shoulders squarely to the mirror.

## Goals

To develop greater proprioception.

## Modifications

Touch a wall and make movements smaller.

## Variations

Close your eyes for one repetition.

# 16 THE TEASER

Leg Extension, Torso Stability, and Single-Leg Balance

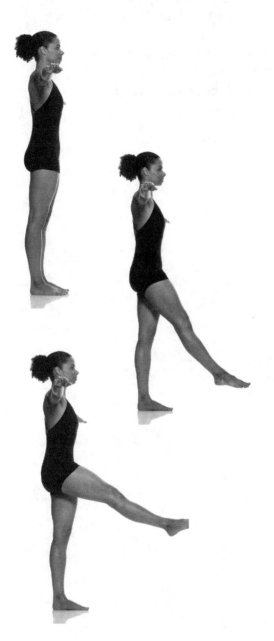

## Level I

Preparation

1. Inhale in the Standing Foundation with arms wide at shoulder height.

2. Exhale and lift the right leg about one foot off the floor.

3. Inhale and lift the foot higher.

4. Exhale to the lower position.

5. Repeat raising and lowering the leg three more times.

6. Inhale and return to the Standing Foundation.

7. Repeat with the left leg.

# Level II

Adds a high leg lift to the side.

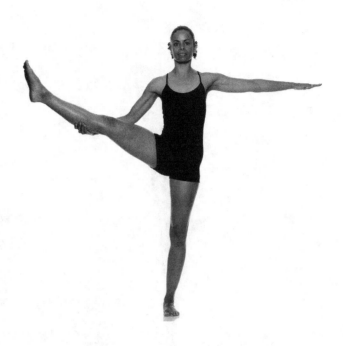

1. Inhale to the Standing Foundation with the arms out to your sides.

2. Exhale to a right Knee Fold and place your right hand behind your right thigh.

3. Inhale and straighten the right knee. The leg reaches to the front of the room.

4. Exhale while shifting the right foot to the side.

5. Inhale to bring the right leg back to the front.

6. Exhale to release the right leg to float down to return to standing on both parallel legs.

7. Repeat with the left leg.

8. Repeat two sets.

# THE TEASER
*(continued)*

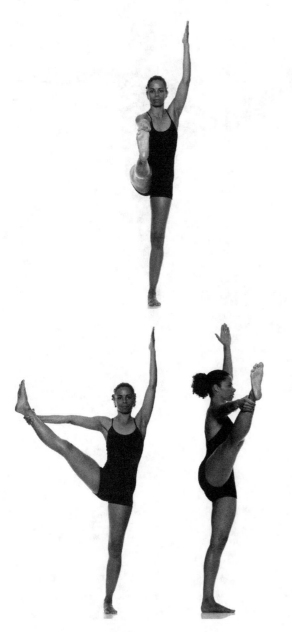

## Level III

Adds arm elevation.

1. Inhale to the Standing Foundation with the arms reaching to the ceiling.

2. Exhale and knee fold your right leg forward, bringing your hand to the big toe (or under the calf).

3. Inhale to straighten the leg forward.

4. Exhale, move your right leg to the right side as you reach your left arm up to the ceiling.

5. Inhale to bring your right leg to the front.

6. Exhale to release the right leg so that it floats slowly back to the floor and return to the Standing Foundation with arms at your sides.

7. Repeat with the left leg.

## Tall Technique

Practice the Single-Leg-Standing Foundation. The weight should be on four corners of the foot. The knee is pulled up and facing over the standing ankle. There is a plumb line connecting the top of your head, your rib cage, your pelvis, and the standing foot.

Don't shift the spine or unlevel the hips to lift the leg higher. Keep the shoulders wide and the spine lengthened throughout the exercise. The spine length in neutral is more important than the leg height. If your spine sinks, your legs can't extend higher.

## Goals

To build leg strength and elongate the hamstrings.

## Modifications

Touch a wall for balance or use a towel to assist the leg lift.

## Variations

Change your focus from the front to the side.

# 17 SWIMMING

Shoulder Girdle Stability with Quick Repetitive Movements

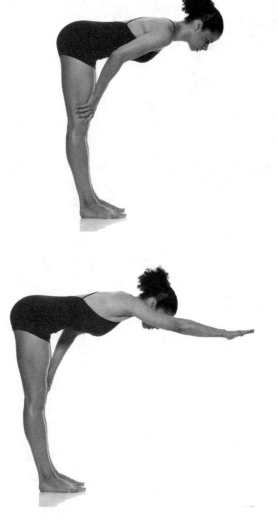

## Level I

Preparation

1. Inhale in the Standing Foundation with your hands on your hips.

2. Exhale, hinge forward at your hips, and slide your hands down your thighs.

3. Inhale and lift the right arm toward the front of the room (in line with the shoulder).

4. Exhale and alternate so the left arm moves ahead in a strong stroke and the right arm returns to the knee.

5. Inhale to lift the arm and exhale to lower it.

6. Inhale to unhinge your hips to the Standing Foundation.

7. Repeat twice.

## Level II

Adds single-leg balance.

1. Inhale in the Standing Foundation.

2. Exhale to widen your back while lifting your arms to the sides at shoulder height.

3. Inhale to slide your right foot backward.

4. Exhale to hinge forward at your hips. Your torso and right leg become parallel to the floor.

5. Inhale to reach your arms to the front.

6. Exhale and bring your hands to your hips.

7. Inhale and reach your arms to the front.

8. Exhale to contract the left standing leg muscles, reaching your arms to the front.

9. Inhale and return to the Standing Foundation and lower your arms by your sides.

10. Repeat with the left leg.

11. Repeat twice.

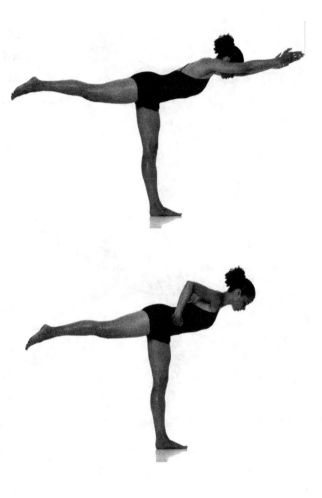

# SWIMMING

*(continued)*

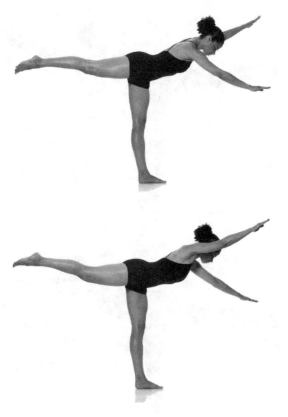

## Level III

Adds arm movements that challenge your balance.

1. Inhale in the Standing Foundation.
2. Exhale to lift your arms overhead.
3. Inhale and extend your right foot backward, keeping the reach of your spine and arms to the ceiling.
4. Exhale to hinge and tilt your body forward over your left standing leg with your arms overhead.
5. Inhale and lower one arm while lifting the other quickly.
6. Exhale and reverse the arms.
7. Inhale to reach your arms evenly to the front.
8. Exhale and contract the standing leg.
9. Inhale and return to the Standing Foundation with your arms by your sides.
10. Repeat with the left leg.
11. Repeat twice.

## Tall Technique

Your shoulder blades follow the movement of the arms by wrapping gently around your side ribs. Keep the shoulder blades wide as you lift your arms near your head. Do not close the space between your ears and shoulders.

Feel how the stability of the shoulder blades lifts the ribs away from the pelvis. Stabilize the torso as you stroke to maintain balance.

## Goals

To challenge balance when your arms move quickly.

## Modifications

Make the stroking movement smaller. Substitute the breaststroke for the arm flutter.

## Variations

Close your eyes in the "swim" phase.

# 18 LEG PULL-BACK

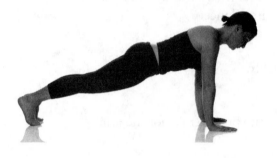

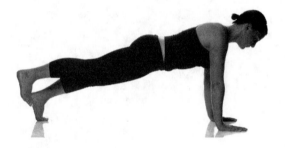

## Level I

Preparation

1. Inhale in the Standing Foundation with your arms by your sides.

2. Exhale, bow, and roll down until your hands reach the floor.

3. Inhale to walk your hands out to the plank position.

4. Exhale and lift the right straight leg two inches off the floor.

5. Inhale to return to the plank position on two legs.

6. Exhale and lift the left leg two inches.

7. Inhale to return to the plank position.

8. Exhale as you lift the leg and inhale as you lower the leg. Repeat the sequence three times, alternating the legs.

9. Exhale to walk the hands back.

10. Inhale to roll up to the Standing Foundation.

# Level II

Adds leg pulses and the pike.

1. Inhale in the Standing Foundation with your arms by your sides.
2. Exhale, bow, and roll down until your hands touch the floor.
3. Inhale and walk your hands out to the plank pose.
4. Exhale while lifting your right leg off the floor and pulse up two times.
5. Inhale and return the right leg to the floor.
6. Exhale to shift your body back to the pike position (down dog).
7. Inhale to return to the plank pose.
8. Repeat with the left leg.
9. Repeat the entire sequence twice.
10. Exhale to walk your hands back to your feet.
11. Inhale and return to the Standing Foundation.

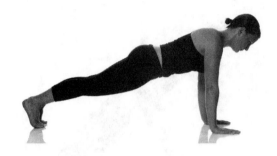

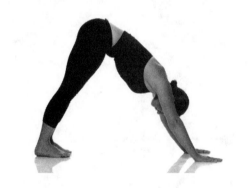

# LEG PULL-BACK
*(continued)*

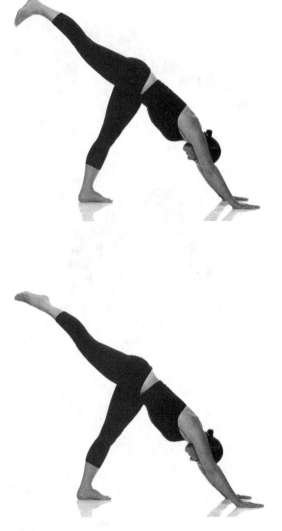

## Level III

Adds arabesque leg extensions.

1. Inhale to the Standing Foundation.
2. Exhale, bow, and roll down until your hands touch the floor.
3. Inhale and walk your hands to the plank position.
4. Exhale, lift your right leg.
5. Inhale and pulse two beats.
6. Exhale and shift back into pike position with your right foot flexed and reaching to the ceiling or an arabesque.
7. Inhale and pulse your right flexed foot upward two beats.
8. Exhale to hold the pike pose with the right leg up in an arabesque.
9. Inhale to return to the plank position with your right leg still lifted off the floor two inches. Place the right foot on the floor.
10. Repeat with the left leg.
11. Repeat two more sets of the entire sequence.
12. Exhale to walk back.
13. Inhale and roll up to standing.

## Tall Technique

Engage your arms from your shoulder blades. Feel the front ribs move into the back ribs. Focus on the exhale and the inhale as you move.

## Goals

To build strength.

## Modifications

Instead of the plank pose, go on all fours with your weight on your knees and hands.

## Variations

In the plank pose go to releve on the supporting foot and rock back and forth before moving to the pike (Level II). Repeat six times releve on the supporting foot in arabesque (Level III).

# 19 THE TWIST

Complex Movements with Rotation, Flexion, and Extension

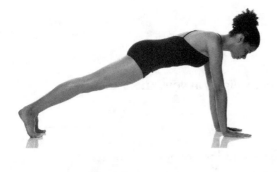

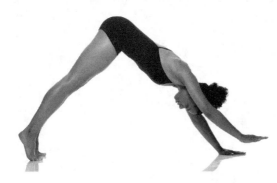

## Level I

Preparation

1. Inhale in the Standing Foundation.
2. Exhale, bow, and roll down.
3. Inhale to walk out to the plank pose.
4. Exhale and move to the pike position.
5. Inhale and lift your right arm off the floor.
6. Exhale to return the right arm to the floor.
7. Inhale to go back to the plank position.
8. Exhale and move to pike.
9. Inhale and lift your left arm off the floor.
10. Exhale to return the left arm to the floor.
11. Inhale, returning to the plank position.
12. Repeat steps 3 to 11 three times.
13. Exhale to walk your hands back to your feet.
14. Inhale to roll up to the Standing Foundation.

# Level II

Adds rotation.

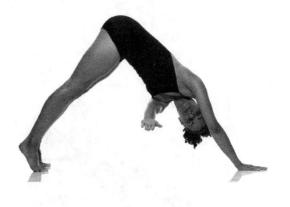

1. Inhale in the Standing Foundation.
2. Exhale while bowing to roll down.
3. Inhale and walk to the plank position.
4. Exhale to the pike position.
5. Inhale to lift your left arm and reach it across the body between your right arm and right foot.
6. Exhale to untwist your spine and place your left hand on floor.
7. Inhale to the plank position.
8. Exhale to the pike position.
9. Repeat on the right side.
10. Repeat twice.
11. Exhale to walk your hands back to your feet.
12. Inhale to roll up to the Standing Foundation.

# THE TWIST
*(continued)*

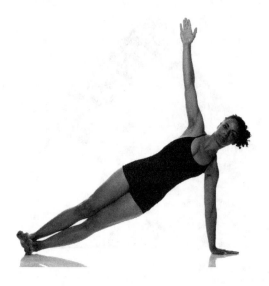

## Level III

Adds side arm balance.

1. Inhale in the Standing Foundation.
2. Exhale and bow to roll down.
3. Inhale to the plank pose.
4. Exhale to shift your entire body to the left hand into a side arm balance, reaching your right hand to the ceiling, with your weight on your left hand and the outside of your left foot (your right foot is stacked on top of the left foot).
5. Inhale, press your hips into the pike position, and thread your right arm across your torso. Your spine and hips pivot.
6. Exhale to return to side arm balance.
7. Inhale to the plank pose.
8. Repeat on the right side.
9. Repeat the entire sequence twice.
10. Exhale and walk your hands back to your feet.
11. Inhale to roll up to the Standing Foundation.

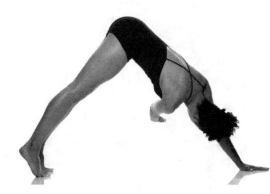

## Tall Technique

The twist is a complex movement involving flexion, extension, and rotation. Focus on each weight-bearing change on two points to four points, then shifting to three points. Connect the lift of your center with upper and lower body motions.

## Goals

To challenge everything.

## Modifications

The feet are scissored.

## Variations

In a right-side balance, cross the left foot in front of the right, then move into the pike position.

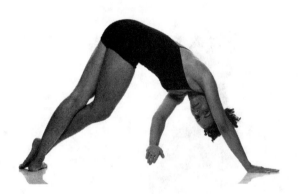

# 20 KICKS
Movement Fluidity in Single-Leg Balance

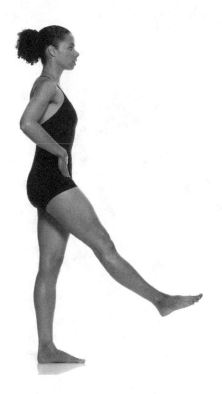

## Level I
Preparation

1. Inhale and stand in the turn-out posi-tion with your hands at your hips.

2. Exhale as you kick forward with your right foot and press down your left stand-ing leg.

3. Inhale to return the right foot to standing.

4. Exhale, then inhale to repeat two more times.

5. Exhale and engage the right standing leg to kick your left foot forward.

6. Inhale to return the left foot to the turn-out position.

7. Exhale, then inhale to repeat two more times.

8. Inhale and stand in the turn-out posi-tion, then exhale to releve. Bring the legs to the parallel position. Descend slowly from the releve while lifting your upper body higher.

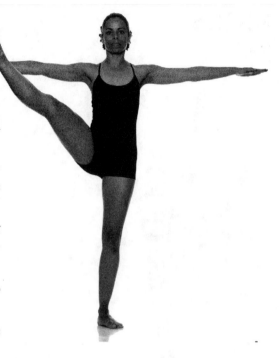

# Level II

Adds arms at shoulder height and diagonal kicks.

1.  Inhale and stand in the turn-out position with your arms reaching out to the sides of the room at shoulder height.

2.  Exhale as you kick to the side with your right foot and press down your left standing leg.

3.  Inhale to return the right foot to standing.

4.  Exhale, then inhale to repeat two more times.

5.  Exhale and engage the right standing leg to kick your left foot to the side.

6.  Inhale to return the left foot to the turn-out position.

7.  Exhale, then inhale to repeat two more times.

8.  Inhale and stand in the turn-out position, then exhale to releve. Bring the legs to the parallel position. Descend slowly from the releve while lifting your upper body higher.

# KICKS
*(continued)*

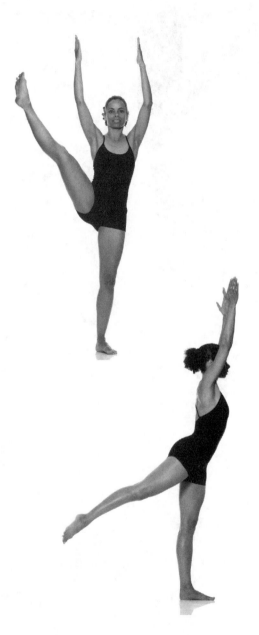

## Level III

Adds arms overhead and backward kicks. It is the same sequence as Level II, but the arms are raised overhead in a V position. And after the diagonal kicks, shift to kick each leg backward. For this kick, keep your back leg turned out with your foot pointed.

1. Inhale and stand in the turn-out position with your arms reaching overhead.

2. Exhale as you kick to the back with the right foot.

3. Inhale and return the right foot to standing.

4. Exhale, then inhale to repeat two more times.

5. Repeat on the left side.

## Tall Technique

Imagine you are kicking a pile of feathers into the air. Keep the standing leg and spine quiet as the other leg kicks. With each kick reinforce the arm connection to keep the spine lifted while the pelvis remains over the standing foot.

With practice, the leg will move higher as you are able to maintain a neutral spine and coordinate the actions. If you kick your leg but bend at the waist or hike your hip, you can't audition for the Rockettes.

## Goals

To maintain Single-Leg Foundation with a lengthened spine as your leg kicks higher.

## Modifications

Touch a wall.

## Variations

Releve and kick front for one repetition.

# 21 PUSH-UP

Torso, Leg, and Arm Strength and Stability

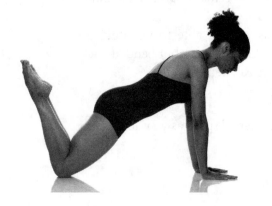

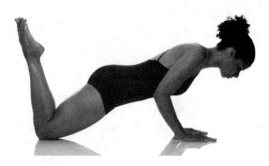

## Level I

Preparation

1. Inhale in the Standing Foundation with your arms at your sides.

2. Exhale, bow, and roll down until your hands reach the floor.

3. Inhale into the plank position with your hands wider than shoulder width.

4. Exhale, bend your knees, and bring them to the floor (your toes point toward the ceiling).

5. Inhale to lower your body by bending your elbows out to the sides.

6. Exhale to straighten your arms.

7. Repeat for five push-ups.

8. Inhale, lower your feet to the floor, and straighten your knees while moving into the plank position.

9. Exhale and walk your hands back toward your feet.

10. Inhale and roll up to standing.

# Level II

Adds the push-up in the plank position.

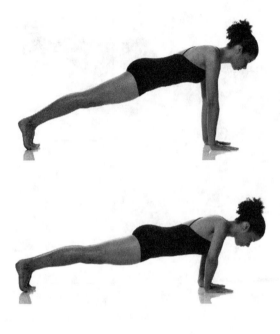

1. Inhale in the Standing Foundation with your arms at your sides.

2. Exhale, bow, and roll down until your hands reach the floor.

3. Inhale into the plank position with your hands wider than shoulder width.

4. Exhale and stabilize the plank position.

5. Inhale and bend your elbows out to the sides.

6. Exhale to straighten your arms.

7. Repeat for five push-ups.

8. Inhale back to the plank position.

9. Exhale and walk your hands back toward your feet.

10. Inhale and roll up to standing.

# PUSH-UP
*(continued)*

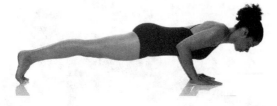

## Level III

Adds a tricep push-up.

1. Inhale in the Standing Foundation with your arms at your sides.
2. Exhale, bow, and roll down until your hands reach the floor.
3. Inhale into the plank position with your hands directly under your shoulders.
4. Exhale and stabilize this plank position.
5. Inhale and bend your elbows into your sides (the elbows stay close to your ribs).
6. Exhale to straighten your arms.
7. Repeat for five push-ups.
8. Inhale back to the plank position.
9. Exhale and walk your hands back toward your feet.
10. Inhale and roll up to standing.

## Tall Technique

Imagine you are a suspension bridge with your feet on one shore and your hands on the other side. Your center suspends your body over water. Your four limbs are equally active.

## Purpose

To build strength in the upper body and triceps.

## Modifications

Practice "push-ups" standing against a wall.

## Variation

Increase the repetitions.

## 22 THE STAR
Challenge Your Mind and Your Body

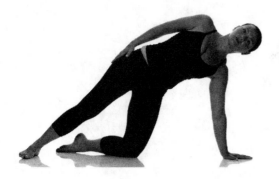

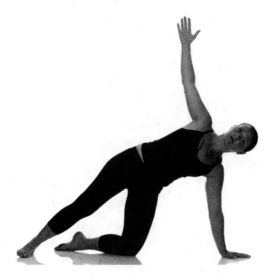

## Level I
Preparation

1. Inhale in the Standing Foundation with the arms at your sides.

2. Exhale, bow, and roll down, bringing your hands to the floor.

3. Inhale to walk your hands out to the plank position. Spread your fingers as wide as possible.

4. Exhale to drop your right knee to the floor and pivot the left foot to the floor.

5. Inhale to reach your left hand to the ceiling, and pivot your hips and shoulders to face the left side.

6. Exhale to lift your hips and ribs.

7. Inhale to return to the plank position.

8. Exhale and walk your hands back to your feet.

9. Inhale, rolling up the spine to the Standing Foundation.

10. Repeat on the left side.

## Level II

Adds leg scissors and side arm balance.

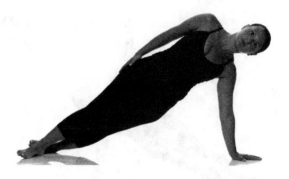

1. Inhale in the Standing Foundation with your arms at your sides.

2. Exhale, bow, and roll down to place your hands on the floor.

3. Inhale and walk your hands to the plank position.

4. Exhale to place your left hand on your left hip and pivot your entire body to side arm balance, with your legs like open scissors (one foot in front of the other).

5. Inhale and reach your left hand toward the ceiling.

6. Exhale with the hips and shoulders facing the left side.

7. Inhale to the plank position, placing your left hand on the floor.

8. Exhale and walk your hands back to your feet.

9. Inhale and roll up to standing.

10. Repeat on the left side.

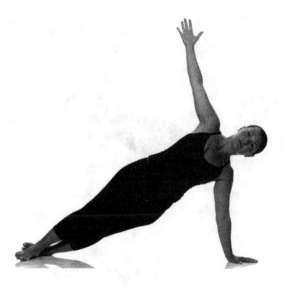

# THE STAR

*(continued)*

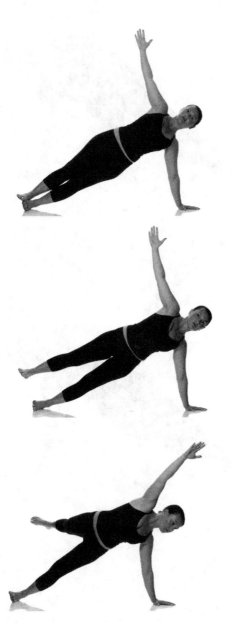

## Level III

Adds arm and leg motions.

1. Inhale to the Standing Foundation with your legs engaged and your entire spine lengthened.

2. Exhale to bow and roll down until your hands touch the floor.

3. Inhale and walk out to the plank position. Your feet are as close together as possible.

4. Exhale, reach the right arm to the ceiling, and pivot onto the outer edge of the left foot into a side arm balance. (The feet are stacked one on top of the other.)

5. Inhale and lift the right leg to hip height.

6. Exhale to swing your right leg back as your right arm reaches overhead.

7. Inhale to swing your right leg slightly forward.

8. Exhale and return the right leg back to the left (stacked).

9. Repeat the leg swings twice.

10. Inhale and return the right hand to the floor in the plank position.

11. Exhale and walk your hands back toward your feet.

12. Inhale and roll up to standing.

13. Repeat on the left side.

## Tall Technique

This is a complex exercise with flexion, extension rotation, and several arm and leg changes. Pay attention to proprioception (where your torso and limbs are in space), focusing and breathing. You should be proud of yourself just for trying this one!

## Goals

To be weight-bearing on two limbs in a side arm balance.

## Modifications

Reduce repetitions on all levels.

## Variations

In Level III transition to plank between the right and left sides.

# 7

# After Standing Pilates

## Sitting (or Half Standing)

During the last few decades we have turned into a nation of flexion addicts. We are sitting at the computer, eating, traveling in cars and planes, eating, watching TV, eating, talking on the phone, and eating. We are sitting, or more accurately, slumping. We are almost always inclined forward even if we are doing nothing. This "posture" degrades our musculature and impacts our neurological systems. In other words, it is bad.

Our bodies are designed to function from a neutral spine. When we are slumped in the sitting position, our muscles become lax. Feel the difference when you sit upright on your sitting bones. Connect the lift of the domes of the pelvis, ribs, and head. Look at your clothes and see how they hang. Now slump and watch how the fabric wrinkles. This is what is happening to your torso muscles. And you wonder why your abdomen is sticking out! Muscles become lax when you slump, so other muscles try to take over the slack of the

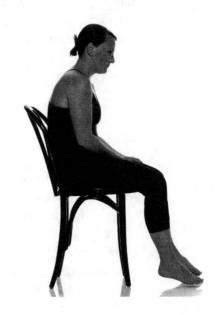

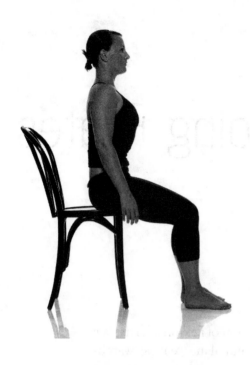

internal support muscles. When you sit for long periods, your hips and shoulders become stiff. Your hip flexors and neck muscles must take up the slack. They are tightening to hold you up. This is not good.

## Crossed Legs

Although slumped sitting is bad, sitting with your legs crossed is the worst possible position. First, circulation is decreased. Second, the combination of compression on one side and overstretching on the other unbalances the spine. With your legs crossed, it is impossible to activate the pelvic floor, and you know now how important this is. If you sit with your legs crossed (and almost everyone does), try this experiment. Put your hands on your pelvis below the navel on your lower abdominals. Sit with a neutral spine with your feet parallel on the floor and feel how the muscle tone increases. Now cross your legs and feel how the tone slacks off. Your spine compensates in this position. The internal obliques are active if you sit on a firm surface, but this activity is greatly reduced when you cross your legs or sit on a soft surface such as a sofa.

## Head Position

So if you have uncrossed your legs, now pay attention to the angle of your head whether sitting or standing. The typical forward head position accelerates aging. The spinal column is the container for the spinal cord. A slumped posture with a forward head changes the flow of signals from the brain down the spinal cord to the rest of the body. Head forward means chin forward, too. This position changes how the signal travels from the spinal cord to the midbrain. This short circuit affects the thinking part of the brain.

# Dynamic Sitting

Since modern life requires a lot of sitting, we need to make it as dynamic as possible. Sit on a chair and position your weight evenly on your sitting bones (under your buttocks) and your pelvic bones (front). This is a neutral position. Immediately you will notice that you are not terribly comfortable. If this is ideal and neutral, then why isn't it comfortable? Your body has become acclimated to a series of bad habits. Reteach your body how to sit. Step one is to change position and avoid sitting still. It is better to *shift between imperfect sitting positions than not to shift at all*. You need to shift just to uncross your leg, then cross the other one. Yes, you know that the crossed-leg syndrome is bad, but this is a habit that is hard to break. Just paying attention to your habit will start the process. Observe that everyone sits this way, even on TV talk shows.

Since you are so accustomed to sitting in the same position, you need inspiration to figure out new positions. Here are some movement ideas.

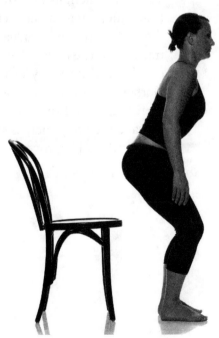

1. Visualize that you can lift the muscles of the pelvic floor off the chair by creating a dome inside your pelvis. Do not squeeze the buttocks or tighten the legs. Put your hands on your waist and intentionally lift the pelvic floor muscles off the chair.

2. Practice lifting any or all of the four domes when you are sitting anywhere, watching TV or in a meeting at work. Or when standing in line. If no one notices, you are probably doing it correctly.

3. Move to the edge of the chair with your weight equally distributed on the pelvic bones. Stay at the edge for a few minutes, then shift back to the center. Then move back in the chair. Stay in neutral for five minutes. Then rest.

4. Lean forward by hinging at the hips with the spine in neutral. Shift your

weight off the chair with your legs. You will be in a squat position. Keep the weight equally distributed on the four points of your foot. Using only your legs and pelvic foundation, rise to standing. Squat, keep the spine long, and sit down again, but use only your legs and feet.

5. Do sitting pelvic moves. Rock back and forth on the chair with your spine elongated. The spine will move from flexion as you rock back on your sitting bones to extension or forward onto the front of the pelvis. This can feel really good.

6. Do the Head Float Fundamental anywhere: sitting, standing, and lying down. It will lengthen the top of your body; then you will look thinner.

7. Knee fold when no one is looking. This feels great, but make sure the chair does not fly away.

8. All of the arm movements—arms circles, rib cage arms, spinal arms— are useful and practical anywhere. Just don't hit anyone.

The Fundamentals and the Foundations are physical and mental exercises. Learn them, remember them, and use them. They retrain the brain to move the body correctly. Gradually new muscle memory is formed. This awareness transfers to the body.

You can do many of the standing exercises anywhere dressed in street clothes. Of course, just standing on one leg and working to align your body with length and space is exercise. Trust me: if you reduce the actions that degrade the body, such as slumping, and add better mechanics, the body will cooperate and improve.

# Afterword

Today Pilates is well-known and appreciated, but only ten years ago attitudes ranged from ignorance to indifference to resistance. A personal story illustrates this change. In 1992 I had a vanity license plate that read "PILATES." Up to the mid-nineties I was often approached by people in parking lots asking me why I had a religious name on my license plate. By 1996 the comments changed to indicate that Pilates was a form of exercise, although exactly what type of exercise was unclear. By 2000 people approached my car while I was stopped at traffic lights seeking recommendations for good Pilates teachers.

This massive shift in favor of Pilates and body/mind exercise has been an exhilarating, albeit bumpy ride due to trademark battles and the "overnight" popularity after decades of obscurity. Now that Pilates is available, we know that it will continue to evolve.

Standing Pilates is what we believe Joe would have created because he always responded to the changing needs of bodies. It was inspired by Joe's favorite quote from the German writer Friedrich Schiller, who said, "It is the mind itself which builds the body."

# Pilates and the PhysicalMind Institute

The PhysicalMind Institute was started in 1991 in Santa Fe and was called the *Institute for the Pilates Method*. It was the first membership and training organization for professionals who wanted to certify in the Pilates method. At that time, there were about one hundred Pilates teachers in the world. By 2004 there were several thousand, and PhysicalMind had become the largest certifying organization in the United States. The institute has a worldwide membership of teaching professionals. It offers a teacher training and certification program in The Method Pilates.

Joseph Pilates came to the United States from Germany in 1926. He was of Greek parentage, but he had lived in Germany since his birth in 1881. The story was that he was small, asthmatic, weak, and friendless. He sought refuge in physical culture and developed his body so that he could defend himself. He arrived in the United States with a new wife, Clara, whom he met on the ship on the way.

Pilates opened a studio on Fifty-eighth Street and Eighth Avenue in New York City. At that time, and until the late sixties, there was no exercise industry in the United States. Health clubs, working out, exercise machines, and routines came of age in the seventies. Prior to that time, Americans did not do formal exercise. Most people were of normal weight. Fitness was a direct response to eating too much, then needing to burn off the fat with aerobics.

Today people seeking body conditioning know that Joseph Pilates led us to bodymind integration. The exercises and equipment that he designed are now finding a large audience because conventional programs have failed.

The Method Pilates works the deeper muscles to achieve efficient and graceful movement, improve alignment and breathing, and increase body awareness. These exercises deliver stretching and strengthening simultaneously in a nonimpact balanced system of bodymind exercise.

In the early days, the Pilates studio struggled until George Balanchine and Martha Graham discovered it. Pilates attracted dancers, and after a while, physical culture buffs and a small elite clientele of avant garde New Yorkers. Pilates died in 1967 at age eighty-eight without any recognition or success. In 1950, very discouraged, he said that he would not be understood for fifty years, and this has proved to be correct.

Pilates is the number one trend in fitness today. The PhysicalMind training programs are offered in certifying studios throughout the United States. There are also certifying studios in Canada, Brazil, Israel, Greece, New Zealand, and Hong Kong. (England, Australia, Argentina, and Colombia will be added in 2005.) In addition to serving a consumer clientele, these studios offer our certification courses. For more information see the PhysicalMind Web site at www.themethodpilates.com.

# Osteoporosis and How Pilates Can Help

O steoporosis refers to porous bones that were once strong and have become fragile as a result of mineral metabolism disturbances and nutritional imbalance. Because there is no physical sensation, osteoporosis has been labeled a silent disease and can cause bone fractures during normal activities such as bending over or during exercises where flexion of the spine is a common movement. There are 1.5 million fractures yearly due to osteoporosis of the hip, spine, and wrist. Approximately 30 percent of all women in the United States over age fifty will experience a spinal fracture, either a vertebral compression fracture or a vertebral crush fracture.

Osteoporosis is *not* a natural result of aging. It is natural to lose some bone tissue in the aging process due to reduced calcium absorption efficiency. Approximately 1 percent of spinal bone loss per year begins around age thirty-five in women, increasing to 3 percent or more once menopause begins, then declining to about 1 percent loss per year after six to ten years. According to studies at the Mayo Clinic, women can lose up to 47 percent of their bone density from the spine during their lifetime, whereas men typically lose about 14 percent.

Early preventive steps include the building of strong bones during childhood and adolescence. This is the best defense against developing osteoporosis later in life. In mature adulthood, strategies to prevent osteoporosis include balanced nutrition; a lifestyle without smoking or excessive consumption of alcohol; moderate physical activity, particularly weight-bearing exercises, strength training, balance, and coordination activities; bone density testing; and medications when appropriate. Standing Pilates is one of the best physical methods to increase bone density. Standing on one leg in women equals a weight-bearing force of four times one's body weight.

## Osteoporosis Categories

Osteoporosis is classified according to the causes of bone loss:

1. Osteopenia, an osteoporosis risk factor, can be congenital or acquired and sometimes exists in people who never reached peak bone mass. It is a condition of low bone mass and may or may not be a precursor to osteoporosis. Some who have osteopenia never get the disease.

2. Primary osteoporosis, postmenopausal, or type I osteoporosis, is rapid bone loss caused by estrogen deficiency and affects the trabecular bone, especially in the spine and wrist.

3. Senile or type II osteoporosis is bone loss in the cortical areas as well as the trabecular areas and progresses more slowly than post-menopausal osteoporosis. It occurs in both women and men around age seventy or older. Fractures of the hip are most common, as are vertebral fractures (wedge type), proximal humerus, tibial, and pelvic fractures. A dorsal kyphosis or dowager's hump is a clinical feature. Calcium and vitamin D deficiency, along with estrogen depletion and age-related changes in the skeleton, are some of the causative factors.

4. Idiopathic osteoporosis can affect youngsters around the time of puberty as well as adults. Its causes are unknown.

5. Secondary osteoporosis.

Medical conditions associated with bone loss in men and women include

- Malignancy (of any type)
- Early oophorectomy (removal of the ovaries)
- Hypogonadism (decreased testosterone in men)

- Spinal cord injury
- Breast and other cancers
- Blood and bone marrow disorders
- Anorexia nervosa or exercise-induced amenorrhea (acquired sex hormone deficiency)
- Turner's or Klinefelter's syndrome (genetic sex hormone deficiency)
- Cushing's syndrome (overactive adrenal glands)
- Hyperparathyroidism (overactive parathyroid glands)
- Hyperthyroidism (overactive thyroid glands)

## Pharmacological Agents That Increase Osteoporosis Risk

- Glucocorticoids such as cortisone, prednisone, and methylprednisolone (for conditions such as asthma, multiple sclerosis, rheumatoid and osteoarthritis, Crohn's disease, ulcerative colitis, lupus, psoriasis and severe dermatitis, liver, kidney, and lung diseases, inflammation and diseases of the eye; also taken in combination with other medications for organ transplants and cancer)
- Thyroxine (principal thyroid hormone; its synthetic form is used to treat hypothyroidism)
- GnRH analogs used in the treatment of endometriosis
- Anticonvulsants, antiseizure medications (hypnotics and barbiturates)
- Loop diuretics (fast-acting diuretics such as furosemide)
- Heparin (long-term) used in the prevention of blood clotting
- Aluminum-containing antacids for gastrointestinal discomfort (prevent calcium deposition)
- Cholestyramine to control cholesterol levels (decreases vitamin D absorption)
- Methotrexate used in the treatment of cancer, immune disorders, and psoriatic arthritis (has toxic effect on bone-forming cells and may alter kidney function, leading to increased calcium loss in the urine)

# Why Bones Change

Bones grow and change throughout our lives, influencing and being influenced by our functional choices. During childhood, adolescence, and early adulthood when the skeleton is being formed, bone formation occurs at a faster rate than bone resorption (removal or loss of bone). Bone remodeling describes the constant process of old bone being removed and new bone being laid down. Osteoclasts are special cells involved in bone resorption (removal) and osteoblasts are involved in cell formation.

Hormones, exercise, and calcium are some of the important factors responsible for the bone remodeling process. The skeleton reaches its maximum bone mass (amount of bone tissue) and density (how tightly the tissue is packed) between the ages of twenty and thirty, after which bone removal begins to occur at a faster rate in both men and women. There is a window of opportunity to accrue peak bone mass during the pubertal growth spurt, which can buffer the amount of bone loss during adult years. Adequate nutritional intake, appropriate circulating hormones, and exercise are necessary for the bone mass to increase during the two or three years of the adolescent growth spurt (genetics also plays a major part). In the mature adult, bone formation and bone resorption continue at equal rates; bone density remains the same as long as these processes are in balance.

Calcium is used to maintain appropriate blood mineral levels, and nerve and muscle function. When the body has an insufficient supply of this key mineral (or the ingestion of calcium and phosphorus is not balanced), it pulls calcium from the bones, which leads to accelerated loss and eventually osteoporosis.

Men begin to lose bone mass at the same rate as women around age sixty-five, when production of testosterone decreases (hypogonadism). Two million men in the United States age fifty and older already have osteoporosis. As a result, they can suffer painful spinal and hip fractures as women do, only at a later age. Alcoholism, chronic kidney, lung, or gastrointestinal disease, calcium deficiency, physical inactivity, long-term glucocorticoid use, and some treatments for prostate cancer, hyperparathyroidism, and myeloma make men susceptible to osteoporosis.

Pregnancy-associated osteoporosis is rare. If it occurs, it is usually identified in the third trimester or postpartum. It is not clear if this disorder is due to the pregnancy itself or to some preexisting condition (caused by heparin or glucocorticoid use). Genetic factors may also play a role. Some women may experience back pain, loss of height, and vertebral fractures. Physiological changes during pregnancy that protect bone include:

- Increased intestinal absorption of calcium, especially in the second and third trimesters
- Increased total vitamin D levels in response to fetal demands
- Third-trimester estrogen surge
- Increased bone loading due to weight gain

Physiological causes of bone loss during lactation include

- Increased calcium demand from maternal bone (varies depending on amount of bone mineral produced and duration of lactation)
- Elevated prolactin (pituitary hormone) levels
- Hypoestrogenic state (reduced estrogen levels)

Bone loss tends to be temporary, and full recovery of density occurs approximately six months after weaning.

Once menopause has set in around the ages of forty-five to fifty-five, women begin to lose bone very rapidly due to the sharp decline in estrogen production by the ovaries. Among other functions, estrogen is a hormone that has a protective effect on bone. It improves absorption of calcium and decreases the amount of calcium lost through urine. Levels decline long before actual menopause is reached. Ovarian production of estrogen may have slowed down five to ten years before true menopause (cessation of menses for a full year). Diagnosis of perimenopausal and premenopausal symptoms could be key in discouraging further bone loss, yet they are often overlooked by doctors and are unknown to most patients.

Perimenopause, the time before and after menopause, involves endocrine changes and certain signs and symptoms associated with the normal physiological event of menopause. There may be a change in the menstrual flow, including heavier periods or more irregular bleeding. Women report increased fatigue, mood swings, and other emotional changes. When a woman has not had her period for one full year, she is said to have gone through menopause, which can be verified by a blood test. The factors determining the menopausal experience are varied and complex. Cultural values, genetics, diet, age at menopause, marriage, menarche, number of children, stress level, and a woman's attitude about menopause may contribute to the considerable variation in reported symptoms.

## Who Is at Risk?

Recent studies show that the average age of menopause (now fifty-two years) is dropping and that many American women start to lose estrogen beginning at age forty. Vigorous exercise and an unhealthy diet can stop menstrual periods and cause some women in their twenties to have bone mass as low as women in their eighties.

Over 28 million Americans, 80 percent of whom are women, are affected by osteoporosis, including 50 percent of women over sixty-five. It is estimated that among men and women over forty-five, osteoporosis is responsible for over 1.5 million bone fractures each year.

High risk factors for osteoporosis include:

- Female of Caucasian or Asian race
- Family history of osteopenia or osteoporosis
- Small frame size or underweight
- Late age at menarche with interrupted cycles (in the United States, average age for start of menstrual cycle is 12.5)
- Amenorrhea or oligomenorrhea
- Women who have never given birth (nulliparous)
- Menopause before age forty-five, either naturally or from surgical removal of ovaries
- Early (before age forty) menopause (average age in the United States is fifty-two)
- Sedentary, or excessive exercising
- Smoking
- Fad or yo-yo dieting
- History of bone density–reducing drugs (heparin, prednisone, synthroid, etc.)
- History of chronic disease, organ transplantation, cancer, overactive thyroid or parathyroid gland, seizures, endometriosis, etc.

- Inadequate calcium and vitamin D intake
- High intake of animal protein, caffeine, alcohol, soft drinks, sodium, sugar, and fiber
- Low testosterone levels in men

Low risk factors include:

- Male gender or female of Hispanic, African-American, or Mediterranean race
- No family history
- Large frame size or slightly overweight
- Early age at menarche with normal cycles and no amenorrhea
- Have had one or more children
- Uterus and ovaries intact
- Late onset of menopause (in fifties)
- Physically active at least three to four times per week for forty minutes
- Good posture and body mechanics
- No smoking
- No fad diets
- No use of drugs that accelerate bone loss (glucocorticoids, antiseizure medications, antacids containing aluminum, diuretics)
- No history of chronic kidney, lung, or gastrointestinal disorders
- Adequate intake of calcium and vitamin D
- Moderate or low intake of animal protein, sodium, sugar, and fiber
- None or low intake of alcohol, soft drinks, and caffeine

## Web Sites

The following Web sites are good sources of information for anyone wanting to learn more about osteoporosis and other conditions that can be improved by engaging in mind-body exercise.

CalciumINFO
www.calciuminfo.com

Colorado Osteoporosis and Bone Disease Center
www.coloradohealthnet.org

Foundation for Osteoporosis Research
www.fore.org

iVillage
www.ivillage.com

Massachusetts Prevention Center
www.preventioncenter.org

Mayo Health Clinic
www.mayohealth.org

Medscape
www.medscape.com

Merck Osteoporosis
www.merck.com/disease/osteoporosis

National Institutes of Health
www.osteo.org

National Institute on Aging
www.nih.gov/nia

National Library of Medicine
www.nlm.nih.gov

National Osteoporosis Foundation
www.nof.org

National Women's Health Information Center
www.4woman.org

Osteo Information
www.osteoporosis.com

Osteoporosis Info (Canada)
www.osteoporosis.ca

P/S/L Group—Doctor's Guide to the Internet
www.pslgroup.com

# Testimonials on Standing Pilates

During thirteen years of teaching Pilates, I have seen many of my long-term clients progress in ways they could not imagine. But not until the standing work was developed by the PhysicalMind Institute did they truly have a sense of their bodies in relationship to the space around them. They are now more confident and secure in knowing what their bodies can do once they leave the studio.

> Leslie Golub
> Leslie's Total Fitness
> Chicago

Joseph Pilates imagined his work to "fit you for life!" Standing Pilates brings his work full circle, off the mat and to the vertical. There is no doubt that Joseph would have designed it himself!

> Lonna Mosow
> Center for Mind Body Fitness
> Eden Prairie, MN

Standing Pilates is the missing link. It is like a baby learning to crawl, walk, and run. The standing work really glues the concept of the Method together.

Sophie Cannonier
Bermuda Integrative Health Co-op Ltd.
82 South Shore Rd. (Nautilus House)
Warwick, Bermuda

Standing Pilates open leg rocker exercise is great for a golfer's conditioning. It improves posture at the address phase, weight transfer, and balance part of the swing.

Charlotte Addington-Weikel
B-Fit Center
Tampa, FL

Standing Pilates is a great way to refocus your workouts and shake up a routine that may have become stale.

Maria Leone
Bodyline Fitness
Los Angeles, CA

The PhysicalMind Institute's transformation of the classic Pilates mat work into standing exercises truly integrates strength, grace and balance in a way that completes the "aesthetic" of the Pilates Method.

Melanie Johnson
Powerflow Pilates
New Haven, CT

The Pilates work on the equipment is invaluable, but clients realize their weakness in balance and standing muscles. I can see why so many seniors have difficulty getting around. This work will make them more mobile and independent.

Cynthia Clark
Thinking Body
Charlottesville, VA

Standing Pilates has been the missing link for clients who are full-time Pilates students. The weight-bearing work helps them get stronger at a faster pace and organizes muscles to function at a higher level. They now perform the other Pilates exercises with greater ease and enjoyment.

Elizabeth Gillies
Inside Scoop
Plainview, NY

Standing Pilates is functionally brilliant; a sedentary population at work and home, young and old, need to remember how to *balance* better on their legs, *concentrate* better up on their feet, and *breathe* better while articulating their limbs in standing.

Nicole Perkovich
Sanctuary 7, The Studio
Miami, FL

Standing Pilates work gives athletes the opportunity to develop an even greater level of coordination, balance, and strength to enhance their performance and prevent injury.

Tom McCook
Center of Balance
Mountain View, CA

Standing Pilates gives proprioceptive feedback faster than the floor work. The client learns where they are in space to maintain correct alignment. This takes their body awareness to the next level.

Katrina Foe
Personalized Pilates
Phoenix, AZ

In the 21st century with an aging obese population the Pilates mission is to restore postural integrity; teach functional movement skills; and relieve pain. Standing Pilates is the fastest way to attain these goals, and, to look slimmer instantly.

Barbara Sampson
Institute Teacher Trainer and Tester

One's body is truly muscularly balanced, when one performs the standing workout with ease.

 Artemis Papakonstantopoulou
 Mind and Body Pilates, Greece

Dancers benefit tremendously from accessing the pelvic floor support for more efficient movement as trained in the Standing Pilates exercises.

 Susan Poland Huffman
 Body Wise Studio
 St. Augustine, FL

Standing Pilates gives clients a functional understanding of how to integrate good postural and biomechanical habits into their everyday lives. Clients also enjoy the challenge of using their core control to find and maintain balance.

 Barbara O'Shea
 Shore Pilates Center
 Spring Lake Heights, NJ

The Spine Twist exercise in standing helps my clients to explore the torso action necessary for getting the best out of walking. Wellington is a hilly city where walking is both a challenge and a joy. Using a subtle spine twist action, they can start to enjoy the views without having to catch their breath first.

 Tania Huddart
 Heart and Bones Pilates Studio
 Wellington, New Zealand

The standing work takes Pilates to a new height, literally. Engaging the MethodPilates concepts in the vertical dimension allows the body to transfer the essential information of the mat work into daily locomotive movements and athletic pursuits.

 Zoe Stein Pierce
 Dancescape
 Fort Worth, TX

Standing Pilates exercises are the ultimate way to transfer core stability into functional movements.

 Susan Greskevitch
 Body Harmonics
 Toronto, Ontario

# Certifying Pilates Studios

## Arizona

Katrina Foe
Personalized Pilates
5010 E. Shea Blvd.
Suite B114
Phoenix, AZ 85254
602-750-5799
www.personalizedpilates.com

## California

Josette Lamotte
Beverly Hills Country Club Pilates
    Studio
3084 Motor Ave.
Los Angeles, CA 90064
310-558-6443 (ext. 1)
www.roomtostretch.com

Maria Leone
Bodyline Fitness Studio
367 S. Doheny Dr.
Beverly Hills, CA 90211
310-274-2716
www.bodylinela.com

Thomas McCook
Center of Balance
1220 Pear Ave.
Suite I
Mountain View, CA 94043
650-967-6414
www.centerofbalance.com

Angelina Spector
Mind-Body Connection
5255 College Ave.
Oakland, CA 94618
510-420-0444

## Colorado

Jennifer Ann Reich
Center Strength
1000 S. Gaylord St.
Denver, CO 80209
303-333-6674

Kristin Smith
Steamboat Pilates and Fitness Studio
1104 Lincoln Ave.
Suite 103
Steamboat Springs, CO 80477
970-879-6788

## Connecticut

Melanie Johnson
Powerflow Pilates
319 Peck St.
New Haven, CT 06513
203-776-0566

## District of Columbia

Michael Wright
Body College
4708 Wisconsin Ave. NW
Suite 2
Washington, DC 20016
202-237-0080

## Florida

Susan Huffman
Body Wise Studios
1797 Old Moultrie Rd.
Suite 101
St. Augustine, FL 32086
904-827-1669 (press 4)

Nicole Perkovich
Sanctuary 7
632 S. Miami Ave.
Miami, FL 33131
304-794-2825
www.sanctuary7.net

Charlotte Addington-Weikel
B-Fit Center
3653 Madaca Lane
Tampa, FL 33618
813-908-2348
www.bfitcenter.com

## Hawaii

Lisa Ortega Robertson
On Balance, Inc.
354 Uluniu St.
Suite 202A
Kailua, HI 96734
808-262-2528

## Idaho

Lori J. Head
Reed Gym@ Idaho State University
Pocatello, ID 83209-8105
208-282-4582

## Illinois

Arlene T. Bass
Body Evolve
600 Central Ave.
Suite 305
Highland Park, IL 60035
847-926-8490

Leslie Golub
Leslie's Total Fitness
213 W. Institute Pl.
Suite 303
Chicago, IL 60610
312-751-1256
www.ltfpilates.com

## Indiana

Idrienne Steiman
Integrated Body Inc.
1220A W. 86th St.
Indianapolis, IN 46260
317-208-2929

## Louisiana

Virginia Davis-Maxwell
Wise Body @ Heartsong Pilates
5150 Hwy. 22
Suite A6
Mandeville, LA 70471
985-845-8045

Alyce Morgan Wise
Wise Body Lafayette
201B Travis St.
Lafayette, LA 70503
337-593-9292

## Massachusetts

Jacqueline Drain Cronin
Pilates Essentials
17 Avery Square
Needham, MA 02492
781-453-0117

## Michigan

Suzette Wilson
Real Results Training
21605 Harper Ave.
St. Claire Shores, MI 48080
586-771-5716

## Minnesota

Lonna Mosow
Lonna Mosow's Center for Mind
    Body Fitness
6409 City West Pkwy.
Eden Prairie, MN 55344
952-941-9448

## Montana

Angelie Renay Melzer
Missouri River Dance
613 Park Dr. S.
Great Falls, MT 59405
406-799-6560

## New Jersey

Barbara O'Shea
Shore Pilates Center, LLC
2409 Old Mill Rd.
Spring Lake Heights, NJ 07762
732-282-0600
www.shorepilatescenter.com

## New York

Elizabeth Gillies
Inside Scoop II
371 South Oyster Bay Rd.
Plainview, NY 11803
516-802-8248

Lesley Powell
Movements Afoot
151 West 30th St.
Room 201
New York, NY 10001
212-904-1399
www.movementsafoot.com

Barbara Sampson
Physical Mind Institute
84 Wooster #502
New York, NY 10012
212-343-2150
www.themethodpilates.com

Joy Puleo
Body Wise Pilates
287 King St.
Chappaqua, NY 10514
914-238-8397

## Ohio

Emily Smith
Focused Fitness
207 Thurman Ave.
Columbus, OH 43206
614-449-1667

## Oklahoma

Jill Balch
A Work in Process
2908 E. 15th St.
Tulsa, OK 74104
918-743-1339

## Oregon

Shelly Stephenson
Bodies in Balance
852 SW 21st Ave.
Portland, OR 97205
503-248-4483
www.bibpilates.net

## Pennsylvania

Lynda Lippin
balanCenter Pilates
915 Montgomery Ave.
Suite 105
Narberth, PA 19072
610-747-0170

## South Carolina

Jennifer Gianni
Embodyment S.C.
730 Santee Ave.
Columbia, SC 29205
803-256-2920
www.embodymentstudio.com

## Texas

John T. Gossett
Eastside Studio
3100 Richmond Ave.
#110
Houston, TX 77098-3015
713-526-8043
www.pilatesconcepts.com

Zoe Stein Pierce, B.A., M.F.A., C.M.A.
Dancescape Studio
1701 River Run
Suite 10001
Fort Worth, TX 76107
817-924-4048

## Utah

Erica Isom
Total Body Pilates
1348 S. 2100 East
Salt Lake City, UT 84108
801-792-3452

## Virginia

Cynthia Clark
Thinking Body
335 West Rio Rd.
Charlottesville, VA 22901
434-975-0336

## Washington

Tara Stepenberg
Breathe! Core Connections
508 6th Ave.
Merlino Arts Building
Tacoma, WA 98407
253-861-8349

## Wisconsin

Susan Hogg
Harbor Wellness Center
2711 Allen Blvd.
Middleton, WI 53562
608-821-6501

## Foreign Studios

Elaine De Markondes
De Markondes Centro de Formacao no
    Metodo Pilates
Visconde do Rio Branco 125
Curitiba-Parana, Brazil 80420-060
55-41-323-2753

Margot McKinnon
Body Harmonics
672 Dupont St.
Suite 406
Toronto, Ontario, Canada M6G 1Z6
416-537-0714

Sophie Cannonier
Contrology! Bermuda Ltd.
82 S. Shore Rd.
Warwick, Bermuda WK09
441-236-0336

Artemis Papakonstantopoulou
Mind and Body Pilates Studio
14 Agion Theodoron St.
145 62 Kifisia
Athens, Greece
010-8010-2311

Mabel Kwan
One Pilates Studio
73 Wyndham St.
21/F Winsome House Central
Hong Kong
852-2147-3329
www.onepilatesstudio.com

Tania Huddart
Hearts & Bones Pilates Centre
64 Oriental Parade
Oriental Bay
Wellington, New Zealand
64-4803-3317

Tzeela Tamir
Dror Raz/Susanne Della Center
Yecheeli 5 Neve Tzedek
PO Box 50257
Tel Aviv, Israel 61500
972-8-850-4966

# Standing Pilates Instructors

## Alabama

Debra Wade
2753 Tammerack Lane
Hampton Cove, AL 35763
256-533-6304

Jane Watkins
2174 Meadowood Dr.
Southside, AL 35907
256-442-3533

## Arizona

Lisa Becksted
170 Beaver Creek Dr.
Sedona, AZ 86351
928-284-4370

Tricia Chiappetta
6774 W. Via Montoya Dr.
Glendale, AZ 85310
623-561-5131

Talitha Eustice
1145 W. Edgemont Ave.
Phoenix, AZ 85007-1114
602-493-4861

Ashley Hooker
9252 W. Purdue Ave.
Peoria, AZ 85345
623-334-3323

Shannon Jette
6019 S. 22nd Lane
Phoenix, AZ 85041
602-703-8350

Pami Kowal
4455 E. Paradise Village Pkwy. S.
Phoenix, AZ 85032
602-795-1789

Barbara Zonakis
9244 Aerie Cliff Lane
Fountain Hills, AZ 85268
480-464-1529

## Arkansas

Roxanne Garrison
Eureka Springs Nursing and
    Rehabilitation
235 Huntsville Rd.
Eureka Springs, AR 72632
479-253-2495

**California**

Simone Alexander
4238 Brookwood Pl.
Highlands Ranch, CA 80130

Allison Allen
735 El Camino Real
Burlingame, CA 94010
650-520-9957

Shirley Archer
1520 Sand Hill Rd.
#408
Palo Alto, CA 94304
800-240-6805

Debbie Baker
1200 Creekside Dr.
Folsom, CA 95630
916-983-7641

Angela Balseger
839 S. Plymouth Blvd.
#4
Los Angeles, CA 90005
323-932-0414

Carol Bayly Grant
1103 Johnson Ave.
San Luis Obispo, CA 93401
805-546-3410

Shannon Beaty
624 Indian Oak Lane
#102
Oak Park, CA 91377
818-706-6301

Jennifer Cancio
5320 Calderwood St.
Long Beach, CA 90815
562-597-8944

Karen Christiansen
77 Pine Hill Dr.
Santa Cruz, CA 95060
831-458-1933

Beatrice Cipriano
3960 Carpenter Ave.
Studio City, CA 91604
818-632-5560

Courtney Cook
74-140 El Paso
Palm Desert, CA 92260
760-776-7903

Laurie Dominguez
4269 Via Marina
#5
Marina Del Rey, CA 90292
310-471-1781

Jean Elvin
PO Box 1032
Santa Clara, CA 95052
650-796-4847

Elana Essers
39365 Chalfont Lane
Palmdale, CA 93551
661-947-9279

Sandy Ferguson
2491 Clarksville Rd.
Rescue, CA 95672
530-677-8947

Jennifer Fiskin
1522 El Dorado Ave.
Santa Cruz, CA 95062
831-462-1486

Dana Frick
2653 4th St.
Santa Monica, CA 90405
310-399-0503

Kristine Gianna
2759 Harrington Rd.
Simi Valley, CA 93065
805-582-9769

Kara Giannetto
1125 Ranchero Dr.
#30
San Jose, CA 95117
408-296-4580

Kristy Guglielmana
127 W. Escalones
San Clemente, CA 92672
949-366-6311

Shannon Haik
113 W. Avenida De Los Arboles
#136
Thousand Oaks, CA 91360
805-405-1375

Alana Hunter
1037 Waverley St.
Palo Alto, CA 94301
650-321-0247

Wilda James
1174 Canyonwood Ct.
#4
Walnut Creek, CA 94595
925-938-7119

Patti Joyce
6680 Alhambra Ave.
#137
Martinez, CA 94553
925-890-9539

Jennifer Lee Ho
860 Vista Rd.
Hillsborough, CA 94010
818-375-0571

Hensl Lise
2015 Arbor Ave.
Belmont, CA 94002
650-595-9847

Tamara Love
15255 Francis Oaks Way

Los Gatos, CA 95032
408-358-8048

Sylvia Lum
PO 1609
Millbrae, CA 94030
650-259-9479

Kamrin MacKnight
1102 S. B St.
San Mateo, CA 94401
650-846-5838

Lynette McLaughlin
10130 Donner Trail Rd.
#6
Truckee, CA 96161
530-550-7796

Jaqueline McNeil
957 Emma Court
Rohnert, CA 94928
707-584-3619

Tracey Messner
5387 Paseo Cameo
Santa Barbara, CA 93111
805-964-3381

Elise Modrovich
5340 Wilkinson Ave.
Valley Village, CA 91607
805-445-9099

Jennifer Monical
3141 Bentley Dr.
Rescue, CA 45672
530-613-6038

Sally Monical
3141 Bentley Dr.
Rescue, CA 95672
530-613-6038

Ava Motter
5006 Boulder Lane
Santa Rosa, CA 95405
707-538-4638

Shannon Murphy
818 W. Grant Pl.
San Mateo, CA 94402
650-345-9731

Christine Naish
2708 Clay St.
Alameda, CA 94501
510-865-4733

Ana Padilla
c/o Longevity for Women
26536 Carmel Rancho
Carmel, CA 93923
831-622-7339

Sue Paul
212 Parrot Lane
Fountain Valley, CA 92708-5720
714-593-8347

Francisca Philip
407 Hedgerow Court
Mountain View, CA 94041
650-541-9611

Conni Ponturo
21844 Ybarra Rd.
Woodland Hills, CA 91364
818-888-6296

Donna Quisenberry
148 Rebecca Way
Folsom, CA 95630-4951
916-985-3205

Jessica Ruggles
1562 High Bluff Dr.
Diamond Bar, CA 91765
909-861-3030

Nancy Schmit
450 Poppy Pl.
Mountain View, CA 94043
650-961-3674

Shelli Stein
2834 Chamier
Fremont, CA 94555
510-790-8994

Ofie Tabarez
PO Box 3294
Palos Verdes, CA 90274
310-960-1727

Sarah Theismann
PO Box 1054
Palo Cedro, CA 96073
530-510-6145

Corby Uzel
8630 Lindante Dr.
Whittier, CA 90603
562-236-9030

John Vosler
4237 Kenyon Ave.
Los Angeles, CA 90066
310-390-4462

Anne Marie Weiss
3175 Temple Court
Santa Clara, CA 95051
408-984-5928

Della Whelchel
74643 Gary Ave.
Palm Desert, CA 92260
760-346-3200

Madeline Wilson
11160 Vista Sorrento Pkwy.
E-101
San Diego, CA 92130
858-755-6069

Aggie Winston
4550 Tam O'Shanter Dr.
Westlake Village, CA 91362
805-373-1440

Ana Worthe
6300 Wilshire Blvd.
Suite 950
Los Angeles, CA 90048
310-486-4514

Frances Zappella-Severance
4417 Laro Lane
Yorba Linda, CA 92886
714-996-7913

## Colorado

Michelle Cantor
381 South Locust
Denver, CO 80224
720-261-0254

Sheri Colosimo
1676 Garfield St.
Denver, CO 80206
720-335-3314

Donna Ferguson
2181 W. Ridge Rd.
Littleton, CO 80120
303-797-2368

Laura Foster
12591 Firenze Heights
#2127
Colorado Springs, CO 80921
719-481-8165

Brenda Geisler
50180 Moon Hill Dr.
Steamboat Springs, CO 80487
970-870-0734

Chris Grotfend
c/o Durango Sports Club
1600 Florida Rd.
Durango, CO 81301
970-259-2579

Wendy Murphy
1357 43rd Ave.
Unit 12
Greeley, CO 80634
970-353-9234

Tracy Petzold
7799 Waverly Mountain
Littleton, CO 80127
303-933-0381

Jennifer Schmidt
1715 E. 16th Ave.
Denver, CO 80218
303-388-7672

Emily Smith
PO Box 4231
Breckenridge, CO 80424
970-393-2000

Dana Tredway
PO Box 772914
Steamboat Springs, CO 80477
970-879-3908

Ryan White
23681 Broadmoor Dr.
Parker, CO 80138
720-851-0605

## Connecticut

Fernanda Araujo
45 Post Rd. E.
Westport, CT 06880
203-927-4861

Alina Ordonez
PO Box 18
Riverside, CT 06878
203-359-4991

Laura Pennock
41 Harborview Pl.
Bridgeport, CT 06605
203-335-1987

171

## Washington, DC

S. Kaye Gardner
4339 Massachusetts Ave. NW
Washington, DC 20016
202-237-8211

## Florida

Jana Allman
417 Orchis Rd.
St. Augustine, FL 32086
904-794-7685

Lore Ayoub
936½ 17th Ave. NE
St. Petersburg, FL 33704
727-236-3457

Patricia Baldwin
4354 McGirts Blvd.
Jacksonville, FL 32210
904-384-9275

Michele Berman
17 South Cirus Ave.
Clearwater, FL 33765
727-895-9587

Christine Borchers
19309 Pierpoint Court
Lutz, FL 33558
813-948-4908

Lisa Branson
855 14th Ave. N.
St. Petersburg, FL 33701
727-822-5121

Jennifer Busby
9735 Fox Chapel Rd.
Tampa, FL 33647
727-736-3419

Teresa Cantrell
10012 Yacht Club Dr. S.

Treasure Island, FL 33706
727-367-4368

Rebeca Cardozo-Pfeiffer
202A Sunrise Dr.
Key Biscayne, FL 33149
305-463-9868

Valerie Carruthers
85 Pine Circle Dr.
Palm Coast, FL 32164
386-437-9372

Kim Christou
5525 NW 48th Pl.
Gainesville, FL 32606
352-371-5802

Melissa Dann
2620 4th St. N.
St. Petersburg, FL 33704
727-525-5103

Christine DeVinney
7476 Canford Court
Winter Park, FL 32792
407-678-0332

Aurora Farber
379 10th St.
Atlantic Beach, FL 32233
904-241-3825

Jeannine Findley
1490 Ocean Blvd.
Atlantic Beach, FL 32233-5746
904-249-2057

Linda Gelcich
4819 Okara Rd.
Tampa, FL 33617
727-985-7068

Randall Justice
975 Imperial Golf Course Blvd.
Naples, FL 34110
239-593-5066

Henriette Mantilla
520 Brickell Key Dr.
BH 43
Miami, FL 33131
305-381-8384

Makaira Maranges
18023 Samba Lane
Boca Raton, FL 33496
561-488-0011

Karen Mirlenbrink
330 Promenade Dr.
#207
Dunedin, FL 34698
727-736-9309

Brandy Price
1045 9th Ave. N.
St. Petersburg, FL 33705
727-455-1753

Annette Randall
6401 99th Way
N. Apt. 15A
St. Petersburg, FL 33708
727-319-3860

Natalie Renew
16 Mulvey St.
Apt. 5
St. Augustine, FL 32084
904-819-5456

Lauri Reynolds, B.S. M.S.
1132 45th Ave. N.
St. Petersburg, FL 33703
727-528-1632

Traci Roshitsh-Weems
10701 Cleary Blvd.
Apt. 106
Plantation, FL 33324
954-781-2984

Barbara St. Claire
130 Woodcreek Dr.

Safety Harbor, FL 34695
727-796-2223

Vicki Sullivan
2744 Woody Pl.
Jacksonville, FL 32216
904-996-7319

Valerie Sullivan-Diaz
13968 W. Hillsborough Ave.
Tampa, FL 33635
813-855-7488

Heather Weldon
1117 Pinellas Bayway S.
Unit 105
St. Petersburg, FL 33715
727-864-3242

Joan Williams
12645 Foxbrook Lane
Odessa, FL 33556
813-920-0744

Roberta Zemo
15 NE 11th St.
Delray Beach, FL 33444
561-274-8593


**Georgia**

Cammy Fisher
2256 Central Ave. A
Augusta, GA 30904
706-364-4156

Diane Narron
210 Harvey Rd.
Brunswick, GA 31525
912-265-1066


**Hawaii**

Deborah Kim
3175 Poelua Pl.
Honolulu, HI 96822
808-358-1038

Lynette Matsushima
45-630 Haamaile St.
Kaneohe, HI 96744
808-236-4402

Cristal Mortensen
3671 Diamond Rd. Circle
Honolulu, HI 96015
808-734-3100

### Idaho

Julie Trimble
6090 S. Settlement Way
Boise, ID 83716
208-373-0628

### Illinois

Diane Baker
849 Fountain View Dr.
Deerfield, IL 60015
847-940-1860

### Indiana

Laurie Bowling
5526 Boruff Rd.
Bloomington, IN 47403
812-824-3037

Janet Ojeda
1805 Woodmere Dr.
Valparaiso, IN 46383
219-531-9464

### Iowa

Dee Sasseen
1235 66th St.
Windsor Heights, IA 50311
515-277-6649

### Kentucky

Gloria Lawrence-Rangel
309 N. Main St.
Lexington, KY 24450
859-461-3447

### Louisiana

Cathy Bergeron
8513 E. Wilderness Way
Shreveport, LA 71106
318-503-7425

Donna Dunlop
570 Pipes Rd.
Ruston, LA 71270
318-768-4426

Natalie Olsen
202 Evangeline Dr.
Mandeville, LA 70471
985-792-5102

Melanie Seifert
1578 Pollard Pkwy.
Baton Rouge, LA 70808
225-761-4755

Jennifer Sloan
645 Rosa Ave.
Metairie, LA 70005
504-236-0041

Mindy Stephens
13339 Molly Mellissa
Walker, LA 70785
225-791-6986

Cameron Tipton
PO Box 1741
Covington, LA 70434
985-867-1486

Ann Wilde
39267 Z Oaks Lane
Ponchatoula, LA 70454
985-386-5728

## Maryland

Danette Allen
853 Kings Retreat Dr.
Davidsonville, MD 21035
410-798-1384

Sharon Brady
2006 Groton Rd.
Pocomoke, MD 21851
410-957-3012

Annie Butler
29797 Bunker Hill Lane
Tratte, MD 21673
410-476-9922

Cristina Carrera
4908 Butternut Dr.
Rockville, MD 20853
301-460-2309

Alison Ford
9930 Logan Dr.
Potomac, MD 20854
301-299-0448

Susanna Fulton
1379 Hillbourne Court
Hanover, MD 21076
443-570-7874

Pamela Kahn
4948 Sentinel Dr.
Bethesda, MD 20816
301-320-8080

Patricia Lofthouse
11700 Old Columbia Pike
#414
Silver Spring, MD 20906
240-876-4211

Tanya Neuman
1015 Veirs Mill Rd.
Rockville, MD 20851
240-314-2057

Jackie Novak
1504 Accokeek Rd.
Waldorf, MD 20601
301-292-1766

Jane Opie
1820 Woods Rd.
Annapolis, MD 21401
410-263-4455

Maya Rhinewine
2912 Lindell Court
Silver Spring, MD 20902
301-942-5917

Bonnie Turner
27 E. Patrick St.
Apt. 3
Frederick, MD 21701
301-668-2699

## Massachusetts

Carol Claflin
171 Old Farm Rd.
Leominster, MA 01453
978-537-0981

Jeannie Fabian
194 Broad St.
Weymouth, MA 02188
617-365-5588

Eileen Gay
44 Rockwood Rd.
Hingham, MA 02043
781-749-0486

Cindy Gilman
35 Kennedy Rd.
Sharon, MA 02067
781-784-1143

Evelyn Herman
57 Gilmore Rd.
Easton, MA 02356
508-238-8238

Christina McKay
225 4th St.
Stoughton, MA 02072
781-297-3566

Annemarie McNeil
PO Box 494
Sutton, MA 01590
508-865-0118

Deborah Nam-Krane
461 Arborway
Apt. 4
Boston, MA 02130
617-524-4092

Tara Simpson
53 Central St.
Apt. 2
Somerville, MA 02143
978-667-1634

Ann Sorvino
c/o Stoneleigh-Burnham School
574 N. Bernardston Rd.
Greenfield, MA 01301
413-774-2711

Diane Trainor
18 Rainbow Circle
Peabody, MA 01960
978-532-1737

Sharon True
139 Alford Rd.
Great Barrington, MA 01230
413-528-2465

## Michigan

Nancy Meier
3551 Windemere Dr.
Ann Arbor, MI 48105
734-997-8838

Judith Veliquette
14537 Spirea Dr.

Elk Rapids, MI 49629
231-264-5254

## Minnesota

Debra Dodge
19700 Schutte Farm Rd.
Corcoran, MN 55340
763-416-1388

Terri Elfner
13740 Flagstaff Ave.
Apple Valley, MN 55124
952-431-3035

Elise Harrison
7815 Victoria Circle
St. Louis Park, MN 55426
612-788-3199

Michelle Maher
7965 Riverview Terrace
Fridley, MN 55432
763-783-9973

Linda Nicoli
2280 Melody Hill
Excelsior, MN 55331
952-474-3729

Kay O'Connell
306 E. 6th St.
Northfield, MN 55057
507-663-1580

Shawn Svendsen
1420 Fourth St.
Stillwater, MN 55082
651-439-4332

## Mississippi

Diane Dryja
4510 Conner Dr.
Hernando, MS 38632
662-449-5491

Sara Pyron
5626 Warwick Dr.
Jackson, MS 39211
601-956-6402

## Missouri

Leslie Arbogast
14 S. Taylor
St. Louis, MO 63108
314-371-1341

## Montana

Jan Bimler
1805 4th St. S.
Great Falls, MT 59405
406-727-5975

Jill Heider
900 Council Way
Missoula, MT 59808
406-542-7748

Angelie Renay Melzer
600 Pine Ridge Ct.
Great Falls, MT 59405
406-799-6560

Laurie Snyder
6631 43rd St. SW
Great Falls, MT 59404
406-453-4897

Quincetta Thompson
PO 1865
Helena, MT 59624
406-442-9485

## Nevada

Catherine Kollier
3770 E. Flamingo Rd.
Las Vegas, NV 89121
702-581-6212

## New Jersey

Gina Berta
49 Woodbrook Dr.
Edison, NJ 08820
732-906-2496

Sylvia Byrd-Leitner
10 Mulberry Court
Tabernacle, NJ 08088
609-859-0956

Diane Checchio
128 Harrow Rd.
Westfield, NJ 07090
908-232-6285

Sheri Cognetti
51 Tamaques Way
Westfield, NJ 07090
908-232-9167

Donna DeSimone
105 Shire Dr.
Sewell, NJ 08080
856-582-0491

Jamie Fagan
46 Surrey Lane
Flemington, NJ 08822
908-788-1926

Donna Hansen
176 W. Shore Rd.
Harrington Park, NJ 07640
201-768-0879

Karen Kavanagh
103 Hardenberg Cove
Point Pleasant, NJ 08742
732-892-1650

Jayne Kwiatkowski
18 Region Dr.
Hazlet, NJ 07730
732-588-7348

Sharon McDaniel
18 Sunset Dr.
Howell, NJ 07731
732-915-6077

Anne Marie Peppe
137 Main St.
Helmetta, NJ 08828
732-656-0202

Heather Pezzello
63 Laura Ave.
Edison, NJ 08820
732-549-1699

Rolin San Juan
38B Meadowbrook Pl.
Maplewood, NJ 07040
973-313-0306

Lesley Smith-Langridge
102 Green Wood Ave.
Madison, NJ 07940
973-410-1349

Jessica Toma
617 Union Ave.
Building 1
Suite 11
Brielle, NJ 08730

### New Mexico

Angela Bonacorsi
PO Box 1292
Santa Fe, NM 87504
505-455-7868

Carol Watson-Brand
4317 Hwy. 15
Silver City, NM 88061
505-534-1261

### New York

Helen Andersson
309 W. 107th St.
Apt. 5B
New York, NY 10025
212-665-5125

Virginia Bell
156 Westfield Rd.
Amherst, NY 14226
716-837-1669

Margaret Brennan
c/o Oak Hill Country Club
346 Kilbourn Rd.
Rochester, NY 14618
585-586-1660

Rose Ann Britschgi
PO Box 916
Skaneateles, NY 13152
315-461-6676

Vanessa Campos
1469 Bay Ridge Pkwy.
2a
Brooklyn, NY 11228
646-325-3067

Scott Cantor
Lifeflex Health Club
18 College Rd.
Monsey, NY 10952
845-354-2474

Dale Eisert
954 Glenwood Rd.
W. Hempstead, NY 11552
516-564-4673

Marilyn Gusmano
225 Erik Dr.
Setauket, NY 11733
631-642-0709

Sherrie Hickey
32 Mayfair Dr.
Slingerlands, NY 12159
518-439-4136

Angie Lee
24-14 41st St.
Apt. 7
Astoria, NY 11103
718-545-2132

Lavinia Long
53 W. 106th St.
Apt. 2A
New York, NY 10025
212-242-2400

Michelle Marino
B15 White Hall Department of
    Government
Ithaca, NY 14853
607-255-9079

Denise Miller
25 Royal Oaks Ave.
Middletown, NY 10940
845-386-8086

Deborah Neuberger
PO Box 616
Remsenburg, NY 11960
631-325-1546

Weena Pauly
100 6th Ave.
Apt. Ground Level
Brooklyn, NY 11217
646-418-6399

Lauren Piskin
1725 York Ave.
#11F
New York, NY 10125
212-876-8424

Bonita Quinn
1 E. 21st Street
#3G
New York, NY 10010
212-475-3577

Eugenia Richardson
186 Cloverland Dr.
Rochester, NY 14610
585-899-6739

Janessa Rick
101 W. 23rd St.
#2401
New York, NY 10011
917-353-2412

Karen Roese
56 Hawkins Ave.
Center Moriches, NY 11934
631-874-2352

Diane Terezakis
1 Tuckahoe Ave.
Eastchester, NY 10709
914-237-5518

Meg Van Dyck
439 5th Ave.
Apt. 2R
Brooklyn, NY 11215
718-768-4393

Stacey Zimberg
25 Franklin Blvd.
Apt. 2A
Long Beach, NY 11561
516-431-1937

## North Carolina

Ann Archer
100 John Martin Court
Carrboro, NC 27510
919-942-6320

Jamien Cvjetnicanin
110 S. Knights Bridge
Cary, NC 27513
919-467-4013

Judy Frederick
5403 Eastern Shores
Greensboro, NC 27455
336-282-1248

Cinnamon LeBlanc-Young
130 Turner St.
Southern Pines, NC 28387
910-692-6129

Susan McKibben
895 Rays Bridge Rd.
Whispering Pines, NC 28327
910-949-4677

Julie Mills
Northstone Country Club
15801 Northstone Dr.
Huntersville, NC 28078
704-671-7672

Deanna Smith
26 8th Ave. NE
Hickory, NC 28601
828-324-3186

Susan Wartell
345 N. Pea Ridge Rd.
Pittsboro, NC 27312
919-545-0371

### Ohio

Cea Cohen
2370 Clubside Dr.
Dayton, OH 45431
937-429-9201

Kelly Enigk
37 Creekwood Square
Cincinnati, OH 45246
513-772-4048

Tina Hazel
9209 Candle Ridge Court
Dayton, OH 45458
937-428-5695

Jacklyn Kearns
5847 Windermere Lane
Fairfield, OH 45014
513-829-3450

Kim Marsee
590 Main St.
Groveport, OH 43125
614-836-5608

Elizabeth McFarland
10250 Locust Grove
Chardon, OH 44024
440-285-8787

Tina Munafo
5586 Clearidge Lane
Cincinnati, OH 45247
513-923-4975

Jennifer Peters
Department of Recreational Sports
106 Larkins Hall
337 W. 17th Ave.
Columbus, OH 43210
614-688-3636

Tiffany Rhynard
1708 NW Blvd.
Columbus, OH 43212
614-486-0625

Emily Smith
2808 Leatherwood Dr.
Columbus, OH 43224
614-449-1667

Marie Stitzel
4727 Moreland Dr.
Franklin, OH 45005
513-423-8730

Mary Willis
5251 Longshadow Dr.
Westerville, OH 43081-7827
614-855-2196

## Oklahoma

Elizabeth Barnett
1401 SW 22nd St.
Moore, OK 73170
405-799-9755

Suze Cheever
12112 N. Dewey
Oklahoma City, OK 73114-8305
405-752-1678

Carol Davidson
809 Adams Trail
Edmond, OK 73003
405-348-2043

Ros Elder
5205 S. Yorktown Ave.
Tulsa, OK 74105
918-747-0735

Benna Else
8454 E. Winchester Ave.
Claremore, OK 74017
918-342-4262

Jeanne Franks
3605 S. Sequoia Ave.
Broken Arrow, OK 74011
918-459-9459

Melanie Heffington
2736 S. 138th Ave.
Tulsa, OK 74134
918-437-7904

Marita Pyankov
137 Rob Lane
Edmond, OK 73003
405-844-9264

Taheera Salim
1518 W. Reading St.
Tulsa, OK 74127

Shelly Walentiny
5749 E. 29th St.
Tulsa, OK 74114
918-836-1568

## Oregon

Bettina Brown
2002 12th St.
Hood River, OR 97031
541-386-1211

Linda Chiverton
5758 Lake Shore Dr.
Selma, OR 97538
541-597-4688

Judy Cifuni
16240 SW Autumn Dr.
Aloha, OR 97007
503-649-8014

Nora Collins
PO Box 264
Dundee, OR 97115
503-538-2964

Debbie Crosman
PO Box 325
Nehalem, OR 97131
503-368-5843

Lori Midrano
6406 SE 19th Ave.
Portland, OR 97202
503-236-3243

Annessa Morey
17285 SW Kinglet
Sherwood, OR 97140
503-625-3024

Milt Nelms
2594 NE Hyde St.
Hillsboro, OR 97124
503-269-5799

Stella Voreas
7906 NW Gales Ridge
Portland, OR 97229
503-203-8407

**Pennsylvania**

Joan Adams
2224 Packard Ave.
Huntingdon Valley, PA 19006
215-938-5044

Megan Armitage
balanCenter Pilates
915 Montgomery Ave.
Suite 305
Narberth, PA 19072
215-307-5166

Lauren Beigle
924 Shady Lane
Bellefont, PA 16823
814-355-5264

Barbara Bruno
51 S. Beech Rd.
Plains, PA 18705
570-822-4064

Lynne Casmay
504 Denton Dr.
Phoenixville, PA 19460
610-935-3494

Misty Cauthen
258 Rainprint Lane
Murrysville, PA 15668
412-387-2671

Maureen Dressman
960 Woodridge Blvd.
Lancaster, PA 17601
717-394-5077

Eileen Erlich
1553 Grovania Ave.
Abington, PA 19001
215-657-6576

Annelise Euler
206 South 13th St.
#505
Philadelphia, PA 19107
215-732-8732

Mary Ewart
Spring and Spiral
5824 Forbes Ave.
Pittsburgh, PA 15217
412-461-9930

Lisa Faloon
734 Clearview Dr.
Verona, PA 15147
412-828-1922

Sabrina Jacomen
1352 Denniston St.
Pittsburgh, PA 15217
412-421-6840

Judy Klunk
112 Murry Hill Dr.
Lancaster, PA 17601-4110
717-560-9282

Bridget Kranson
83 Birch St.
Wilkes-Barre, PA 18702
570-819-1962

Stacey Little
2 Waterview Rd.
N8
West Chester, PA 19380
610-344-9066

Donna Luck
1 Bridge Three Lane
Pipersville, PA 18947
610-294-0101

Joanna McLaughlin
485A Kirk Lane
Media, PA 19063
610-892-4919

Andrea Miller
312 Yorkshire Dr.
Harrisburg, PA 17111
717-540-1506

Sarah Orlowitz
507 Haverford Ave.
Narberth, PA 19072
610-667-7854

Jeff Prall
321 N. Front St.
2G
Philadelphia, PA 19106
215-629-1108

Nadine Quava
67 Fairfax Village
Harrisburg, PA 17112
717-939-0289

Andrea Sapiente
1561 Watson St.
Williamsport, PA 17701
570-745-3139

Carol Rachel Shore
1105 Hower Lane
Philadelphia, PA 19115-4810
215-740-0473

Jill Siegel
367 Harshaw Dr.
Chester Springs, PA 19425
610-458-0618

Amanda Smothers
288 Iven
2A
St. Davids, PA 19087
610-457-0458

Rhea St. Julien
4640 Hazel Ave.
Apt. 2
Philadelphia, PA 19143
215-727-2881

Carol Swanson
708 Galen Dr.
State College, PA 16803
814-234-2317

Jean-Marie Vuk
1450 West Chester Pike
Apt. 650
West Chester, PA 19382
610-344-7710

**Rhode Island**

Elizabeth Giles
215 Pleasant St.
Apt. 2
Providence, RI 02906
401-246-7570

**South Carolina**

Debbie Martin
623 Bluff Pointe
Columbia, SC 29212
803-781-9099

Laura Rogers
116 Greenway Court
West Columbia, SC 29170
803-951-3192

Amy Rosenberg
Cliffs Valley
25 Painters Creek Rd.
Travelers Rest, SC 29690
864-271-4998

## South Dakota

Karla Byrum
604 E. 58th St.
Sioux Falls, SD 57108
605-336-0801

Raena Hillman
1917 Briarden Court
Sioux Falls, SD 57108
605-334-2884

## Texas

Alaina Alexander
2189 Pine Dr.
Conroe, TX 77304
936-524-0314

Charisse Barry
3603 Pemberton Dr.
Pearland, TX 77584
281-489-6251

Monica Bauer
QLS Family Fitness, Wellness
    & Sport
20515 W. Lake Houston Pkwy.
Humble, TX 77346
281-812-6963

Christine Bergeron
2010 Vallejo St.
Austin, TX 78757-2834
512-482-8650

Amanda Blanda
19015 Polo Meadow
Humble, TX 77346
281-852-6648

Jessica Campbell
6138 Abington Way
Houston, TX 77008
713-802-2588

Melissa Cantwell
204 Cedar Lake Dr.
League City, TX 77573
281-554-9974

Kim Marie Cramer
14227 Whitecross Dr.
Houston, TX 77083
281-575-6205

Terri Crayne
6310 Berlinetta Dr.
Arlington, TX 76001
817-557-5667

Stephanie Hahn
7501 Bella Vista Trail
Austin, TX 78737
512-301-8734

Elizabeth Lehmann
1377 County Rd. 676
Dayton, TX 77535
936-258-4738

Debbie Lezama
3511 Pinto Pony Lane
San Antonio, TX 78247
210-402-3316

Sacha Moore
3513 Cordone St.
Fort Worth, TX 76133
817-343-0713

Stephanie Pepi
2002 Forest Park Blvd.
#8
Fort Worth, TX 76110
817-735-1622

Kay Smith
3912 Stonehaven Dr.
Colleyville, TX 76034
817-571-8657

Crystal Titus
5417 S. Mopac
#107
Austin, TX 78749
512-775-5485

Judith Villela
1105 N. 45th St.
McAllen, TX 78501
956-227-0274

Jennifer White
3417 Grandview
San Angelo, TX 76904
325-494-5983

Deanna Young
10718 Lake Winderest
Magnolia, TX 77354
281-356-9848

## Utah

Shauna Beck
2212 Emerson Ave.
Salt Lake City, UT 84108
801-582-1013

Shannon Peay
2172 Emerson Ave.
Salt Lake City, UT 84108
801-698-3096

## Virginia

Pegeen Albig
7625 Cedar Grove Lane
Radford, VA 24141
540-639-3468

Debra Berke
1115 N. Illinois St.
Arlington, VA 22205
703-237-9710

Kathleen Boisvert
11710 Rockaway Lane
Fairfax, VA 22030
703-502-9680

Jane Burgess
20198 Southhampton Pkwy.
Courtland, VA 23832
434-658-4661

Cathy Cannon
2431 Nottingham Rd.
Roanoke, VA 24014
540-343-5238

Beth Copeland
312 W. Bute St.
Norfolk, VA 23510
757-622-9622

Deanna DeVito
1005 Fairhaven Rd.
Chesapeake, VA 23322
757-546-7663

Lucille Dowell
194 Riding Chapel Rd.
Stephens City, VA 22655
540-869-2153

Ella Eavers
129 Shemariah Rd.
Middlebrook, VA 24459
540-887-8404

Pamela Edwards
3272 Wheats Valley Rd.
Bedford, VA 24523
540-586-8790

Erin Garvin
5415 Med Mont Circle
Roanoke, VA 24018
540-989-0434

Melanie Hanson
7848 Crittenden Rd.
Suffolk, VA 23432
757-255-0050

Holly Holland
12905 Westbrook Dr.
Fairfax, VA 22030
703-626-6997

Sheree Kiser
407 College Circle
Staunton, VA 24401
540-886-3823

Alice Krantz
465 Windmill Point Rd.
Hampton, VA 23664
757-851-8452

Gilson Lincoln
1901 Link Rd.
Lynchburg, VA 24503
804-384-2682

Angelique Lockhart
5803 Bunker Wood Lane
Burke, VA 22015
703-425-6873

Helene Matthes
718 Firethorn Rd.
Chesapeake, VA 23320
757-548-8984

Debbie Rackham
12111 Park Shore Court
Woodbridge, VA 22192
703-490-0395

Katherine Shaver
13 Frank Hunt Court
Poquoson, VA 23662
757-868-6000

Terry Smith
1059 Naval Ave.

Portsmouth, VA 23704
757-252-2393

Barbara Spieth
Fox Chase Leasing Office
320 N. Jordan St.
Alexandria, VA 22304
703-823-5138

Gerry Stowers
219 W. Beverley St.
Suite 206
Staunton, VA 24401
540-255-2182

Jolene Swann
511 Willoughby Lane
Staunton, VA 24401
540-294-0221

Jennifer Trauner
421 Sanford St.
Apt. B
Rabford, VA 24141
540-731-5240

Karen Waldron
290 Boner's Run Rd.
Shawsville, VA 24162
540-268-1735

Jennifer Yates
139A Reynolds Dr.
Rustburg, VA 24588
434-528-3119

## Washington

Michele Crane
24645 47th Pl. SW
Vashon, WA 98070
206-463-3755

Candy MacLeod
2835 194th Ave. SE
Sammamish, WA 98075
425-557-2854

Millicent O'Brien
1060 York St.
Apt 204
Bellingham, WA 98229
360-527-1856

Veronica Romey
PO Box 1601
Friday Harbor, WA 98250
360-370-5700

Cathy Schlieman
5609 Walla Walla Lane
Yakima, WA 98903
509-965-0462

Jordan Vincent
26421 SE Duthie Hill Rd.
Issaquah, WA 98029
425-391-5557

## Wisconsin

Connie Cappy
2400 Schafer Circle
Appleton, WI 54915
920-749-1796

Megan Deguire
5034 N. Berkley Blvd.
Whitefish Bay, WI 53217
414-961-3282

Wendy Heldt
2625 N. McDonald St.
Appleton, WI 54911
920-730-8474

Susan Hogg
1535 Red Oak Ct.
Middleton, WI 53562
608-831-1051

Annette Krisko
905 Hanksfield Pl.
Prairie Du Sac, WI 53578
608-644-8212

## Australia

Dana Rader
106/2 Pier St.
Port Melbourne, Victoria 3207
305-931-0958

## Bermuda

Amanda Batista
111 St. John's Rd.
Pembroke HM09
441-295-6839

Caroline Black
7 Astwood Rd
Paget PG04
441-236-3234

Mary Faulkeberry
21 Burnt House Hill
Warwick WK04
441-238-1007

Marisa Hall
1 My Lord's Bay Drive
Hamilton Parish CR02
441-295-5151 ext. 1909

Shirley Hardy
12 Daisyfield Dr.
Sandy MA 05
441-737-0845

Jane Jones
5 Windy Ridge Rd.
Warwick PG01
441-298-3704

Desiree Macleod
20 St. Ann's Rd.
Brenven House
South Hampton SN02
441-238-7354

Carmen Mitchell
PO Box WK 262
Warwick WKBX
441-236-8294

Alexandra O'Neill
9 St. James's Village
Flattes FL04
441-295-9183

Iduma Ortega
Bermuda Integrative Health Co-op
Nautilus House
82 South Shore Rd.
Warwick
441-236-0336

Sandra Penner
82 N. Shore Rd. NE
Pembroke HM13 11
441-292-9253

Ana Slater-Steede
PO Box HM3285
Hamilton HMPX
441-232-0784

Renata Urbanska
PO Box HM2713
Hamilton HMLX
441-293-7342

Margaret Weale
22 Church Rd.
Southampton SN01
441-236-1553

Erica John
c/o Dr. Vincent John, The Arches
13 Berry Hill Rd.
Paget DV03
441-238-4712

**Canada**

**Alberta**

Dianne Anton
204 Grier Terrace NE
#6
Calgary, AB T2K 5Y7
403-730-3827

Helen Cheung
73 Evergreen Close SW
Calgary, AB T2Y 2X8
403-254-0393

Laurie Dawson
433 9th St. NE
Calgary, AB T2E 4K2
403-262-4277

Dorothy Dicks
5019 Norris Rd. NW
Calgary, AB T2K 5R6
403-289-1773

Glory Durnin
196 Sackville Dr. SW
Calgary, AB T2W 0W6
604-251-8130

Jen Huebner
500 5th Ave. SW
Chevron, AB T2P 0L7
403-234-5361

Cheryl Knowles
47-7172 Coach Hill Rd. SW
Calgary, AB T3H 1C8
403-519-6122

Carol Lindsay
82 Edenstone VI NW
Calgary, AB T3A 4T5

Carla Scholten
16 Falsby Way NE
Calgary, AB T3J 1C3
403-285-9516

Cathy Sevcik
437 Ronning St.
Edmonton, AB T6R 1Z2
780-438-4039

Theresa Shaw
3626 67th St. NW
Calgary, AB T3B 4JY
403-268-2205

Travis Thiebeault
8427 Center St. NW
Calgary, AB T3K 1J6
403-275-8289

Anna Wilson
41 Sandalwood Close NW
Calgary, AB T3K 4B4
403-274-1424

Tara Bennett
10736 69th Ave.
Edmonton, AB T6H 2E1

Cynthia Everett
4724 21st Ave. NW
Calgary, AB T3B 0W7
403-202-3681

Teresa Krahn
543 Brookpark Dr. SW
Calgary, AB
403-281-3830

Jeanine Robinson
10 Sierra Nevada Pl. SW
Calgary, AB
403-686-2600

**British Columbia**

Becky Allen
1407 Selby St.
Nelson, BC V1L 2W4
250-352-6684

Pamela Blackmon
21511 87B Ave.
Langley, BC V1M 2E6
604-888-7279

Kimberly Byrne
3685 Argyll St.
Abbotsford, BC V2S 7A9
604-385-4078

Samantha Cramer
103-503 W. 16th Ave.
Vancouver, BC V5Z 4N3
604-731-4950

Rochelle Emnace
193 Aquarius Mews
Apt. 1007
Vancouver, BC V6Z 2Z2
604-809-2431

Ashley Hamilton
1990 Barclay St.
Apt. 307
Vancouver, BC V6G 1L3
604-738-7157

Margie Hardy
4231 Candlewood Dr.
Richmond, BC V7C 4V9
604-275-7374

Monique Hurteau
PO Box 1773
Prince George, BC V2L 4V7
250-964-1120

Pamela Keefe
1855 Campbell Ave.
Port Coquitlam, BC V3C 4T1
604-552-1133

Anne Kerswell
3333 Gibbins Rd.
Duncan, BC V9L 6E5
250-748-5760

Elisabeth Komlosi
1040 King Albert Ave.
Unit 119
Coquitlam, BC V3J 1X5
604-931-1435

Karin McFarlin
3290 W. 4th Ave.
Flat 205
Vancouver, BC V6K 1R9
604-790-7669

Ditta Overgaard
2260 W. 8th Ave.
Suite 308
Vancouver, BC V6K 2A7
604-313-1976

Marge Pollard
107 Pine St.
Nelson, BC V1L 5S5
250-229-4606

Cinzia Toniolo
2406 W. Fifth Ave.
Suite 1
Vancouver, BC V6K 1S8
604-736-6527

Lorna Trent
4326 Birch Ave.
Terrace, BC V8G 4T8
250-635-7342

## New Brunswick

Elizabeth Crabbe
189 Tapley Rd.
Bristol, NB E7L 2E3
506-392-8204

Janet Downey
18 Downey Lane
Valley Road, NB E3L 4V9
506-466-5356

Lindsey Laidlaw-Sweeney
79 Sprucewood Dr.
New Maryland, NB E3C 1C6
506-450-1277

Jan Majerovich
12 McDade St.
Bedell, NB E7M 4P5
506-325-2561

Christy Roy
16 McDade St.
Bedell, NB E7M 4P2
506-328-2442

Lee Saunders
800 Route 885
Intervale, NB E4Z 4Y7
506-756-9008

Zsuzsanna Szabo-Nyarady
825 Aberdeen St.
Fredericton, NB E3B 1S9
506-454-0555

Maggie Vaughan
183 Argyle St.
Fredericton, NB E3B 1T6
506-454-2950

## Ontario

Cristine Adams
4 Wagner Rd.
Ottawa, ON L0M 1P0
705-446-1308

Julie Barban
PO Box 1438
Haliburton, ON K0M 1S0
705-457-4092

Maura Bommer
PO Box 855
Vineland, ON L0R 2C0
905-562-0068

Ahmé Bovee
32 Chillico Dr.
Guelph, ON N1K 1Y8
519-763-0423

Darlene Buan-Basit
100-18 Red Path Ave.
Toronto, ON M4S 2J7
416-545-0498

Georgia Burns
909 Day St.
Apt. 716
Toronto, ON M5S 3G2
647-298-9835

Karen Carew
17 Belton Court
Whitbury, ON L1N 5P2
905-666-9702

Kim Cochrane
213 Walkerville Rd.
Marknam, ON L6B 1B9
905-472-1405

Susan Cocks
334 Mt. Albion Rd.
Hamilton, ON L8K 5T2
905-578-1492

Jennifer Coyne
40 Park Rd.
Apt. 506
Toronto, ON M4W 2N4
416-972-9994

Lori Dunn
97 Douglas Ave.
Toronto, ON M5M 1G4
416-485-5607

Stephen Filipowicz
56-667 Pinerow Crescent
Waterloo, ON N2T 2L5
519-725-5410

Tracy Frohlick
241 Markham St.
Toronto, ON M6J 2G7
416-363-4044

Victoria Gardiner
195 Galaxy Blvd.
Etobicoike, ON M9W 6R7
416-674-7809

Jennifer Geraghty-Gorman
403-161 East Ave. S.
Hamilton, ON L8N 2T8
905-524-0575

Mark Gutkin
176 John St.
Suite 402
Toronto, ON M5T 1X5
416-542-1490

Kristy Hoornick
177 Stepen Dr.
#107
Etobicoke, ON M8Y 3N5
416-239-4169

Jill Jacoby
298 Glenridge Dr.
Waterloo, ON N2J 3W4

Amanda Jeromel
1520 Elm Rd.
Oakville, ON L6H 1W2
905-844-9409

Ana Kokolakis
135 Rose Ave.
Apt. 1408
Toronto, ON M4X 1P1
416-413-9909

Vicki Koutalianos
21 McRoberts Ave.
Toronto, ON M6E 4P3
416-654-4372

Chrystine Langille
Break Out!
2 Mary Gapper Crescent
Unit 24
Richmond Hill, ON l4C 0J4
905-770-8022

Hadar Levac
291 Avenue Rd.
#811
Toronto, ON M4V 2G9
416-961-3273

Tracy Lewis-Currie
5555 Prince William Dr.
Unit 20
Burlington, ON L7L 6P3
905-631-5000 ext. 6351

Lyndsey Linkert
1063 King's St. W.
Hamilton, ON L8S 1L8
352-429-5414

Vera Mader
260 Cedarmere 201
Orillia, ON L3V 7H1
705-326-2894

Jayne Mandic
PO Box 204
Bethany, ON L0A 1A0
705-277-2580

Carol Manning
182 Trail Ridge Lane
Unionville, ON L6C 2C5
401-887-4039

Nancy Martin Recovery Garment
    Center
16 Heintzman Ave.
Toronto, ON M6P 2J6
416-767-6036

Alison McMahon
1315 Silverspear Rd.
Apt. 411
Mississauga, ON L4Y 2W8
905-755-3502

Sue Nash
14 Wood Duck Court
Guelph, ON N1C 1B1
519-763-0066

Dana Radziunas
107 Colbeck St.
Toronto, ON M6S 1V3
416-769-0174

Pamela Robinson
87 Strath Ave.
Toronto, ON M8X 1R7
416-231-1395

Pamela Rooke
1595 Applewood Rd.
Mississauga, ON L5E 2M2
905-271-8001

Louise Saunders
15 Howard Dr.
North York, ON M2K 1K4
416-222-0485

Pauline Shea
38-10 Highgate Dr.
Stony Creek, ON L8J 3P7
905-561-6135

Eileen Sheppard
352 Ball St.
Suite 304
Cobourg, ON K9A 3J2
905-373-8368

Ann Stallman
96 Essex St.
Guelph, ON N1H 3L1
519-821-9389

Denise Lachance Ward
RR2, Highway 7
#8351
Rockwood, ON NOB 2KO
519-856-2717

## Quebec

Myra Aubry
15 De L'epee
Apt. 6
Outremont, QB H2V 3S8
514-276-5912

Tracy Eades
54 Montee Ste. Marie
Ste. Anne de Bellevue, QB H9X 2C1
514-756-9008

## Saskatchewan

Catherine Lavelle-Wicklund
PO Box 245
Milden, SK S0L 2L0
306-935-2244

## Colombia

Maria Clara Ramirez Roa
Calle 86 #764
Apt. 501
Bogota
401-123-67619

## Japan

Keiko Minowa
3-63-6-202 Nishigahara Kitaku
Tokyo 114-0024
81-3-9078459368

## Mexico

Shula Atri Economia
#63 PH11 Lomas Anahuac
Huixquilican Edo de Mexico
Mexico City
C.P. 52760
604-632-0145

## New Zealand

Tania Huddart Hearts & Bones Pilates
    Centre
64 Oriental Parade
Oriental Bay, Wellington
510-594-0545

# Certified Pilates Instructors

## Arizona

Barbara Zonakis
9244 Aerie Cliff Lane
Fountain Hills, AZ 85268
480-464-1529

## California

Cynthia Adams
200 Packet Landing Rd.
Alameda, CA 94502
510-521-5414

Artemis Anderson
583 Belvedere St.
Apt. A
San Francisco, CA 94117
415-566-6625

Liezl Austria
1853 Webster St.
Apt. 6
San Francisco, CA 94115
415-819-2849

Marina Baorni
4181 La Salle
Culver City, CA 90232
310-280-0225

Tracy Bauer
159 Shorebreaker Dr.
Laguna Niguel, CA 92677
949-845-5731

Nicole Bonadonna
Attn: Jethro DeHart
333 Broadway
San Francisco, CA 94133
415-922-9992

Alice Booth
3845 Centinella Dr.
North Highlands, CA 95660
925-786-6400

Yanire Brancato
30414 Rainbow View Dr.
Agoura Hills, CA 91303
818-597-9805

Alana Burton
3338 Scarborough St.
Los Angeles, CA 90065
323-221-7030

Karen Christiansen
77 Pine Hill Dr.
Santa Cruz, CA 95060
831-458-1933

Rosie Cole
2630 S. Fitch Mountain Rd.
Healdsburg, CA 95448
707-431-9861

José Comoda
In care of: The Working Body
614 Grand Ave.
Oakland, CA 94610
415-359-6448

Angela Curran
238 Westminister Ave.
Venice, CA 90291
310-392-1930

Bob DeNatale
472 Duboce
San Francisco, CA 94117
415-864-7020

Elana Essers
39365 Chalfont Lane
Palmdale, CA 93551
661-947-9279

Celi Franke
1431 Manhattan Beach Blvd.
Apt. F
Manhattan Beach, CA 90266
310-798-6599

Elisa Garcia
Sports Club LA
747 Market St.
4th Floor
San Francisco, CA 94103
415-440-3069

Grace Garne
516 Scenic Ave.
San Anselmo, CA 94960
925-680-7716

Jennie Gilman
4211 Wake Robin Dr.
Glen Ellen, CA 95442
707-939-3606

Owen Grady
1135 Madison Ave.
Redwood City, CA 94061
650-839-9980

Cheryl Graves
5633 Farmdale Ave.
North Hollywood, CA 91601
818-985-3901

Sandra Herting
912 England St.
Apt. C
Huntington Beach, CA 92648
714-960-3374

Sarah Hoefer
54 Los Gatos Blvd.
Apt. 2
Los Gatos, CA 95030
408-354-5130

Debra Isaacson
2637 Fransico Way
El Cerrito, CA 94530-1530
510-233-9233

Wilda James
1174 Canyonwood Court
#4
Walnut Creek, CA 94595
925-938-7119

Karyn Kasvin
16 Athlone Way
Menlo Park, CA 94025
650-261-9564

Mike Kazemi
PO Box 427002
San Francisco, CA 94142
415-824-1869

Bliss Kohlmyer
139 Hugo St.
#4
San Francisco, CA 94122
415-970-0060

Hensl Lise
2015 Arbor Ave.
Belmont, CA 94002
650-595-9847

Sheri Long
755 Washington St.
El Segundo, CA 90245
310-640-0088

Stephanie Vannicola Magsanay
1005 Jennifer Meadows Court
Danville, CA 94506
415-922-9711

Natalie Mandrick
11980 Laurelwood Dr.
Apt. 17
Studio City, CA 91604
818-753-4027

Toni Marano
23221 Via Milano
Laguna Niguel, CA 92677
949-249-0606

Melody McKnight
4702 Kraft Ave.
North Hollywood, CA 91602
818-324-6273

Sharon Meister
1071 N. Rodeo Gulch
Soquel, CA 95073
831-476-6313

Michele Melvin
4083 School St.
Pleasanton, CA 94566
925-485-1933

Krista Miller
5051 Klump Ave
North Hollywood, CA 91601
818-404-2154

Elise Modrovich
5340 Wilkinson Ave.

Valley Village, CA 91607
805-445-9099

Kira Morris
7306 Balboa Blvd.
Unit B
Van Nuys, CA 91406
818-505-1973

Christine Naish
2708 Clay St.
Alameda, CA 94501
510-865-4733

Sadie Nutter
1575 Scott St.
Apt. B
San Diego, CA 92106
619-222-0652

Jeannette Opalski
951 S. 12th St.
Apt. 218
San Jose, CA 95112
408-998-8754

Tanya Paiella
131 Hemlock Ave.
Apt. 1
Carlsbad, CA 92008
760-533-6662

Phyllis Perkins
4331 Cognac Court
Loomis, CA 95650
916-652-1184

Gina Petelin
4073 Gresham St.
Apt. 5
San Diego, CA 92109
858-483-6205

Maricar Pratt
30616 Rainbow View Dr.
Agoura Hills, CA 91301
818-879-5064

Christa Rypins
PO Box 62
Murphys, CA 95247
650-964-6540

Jocelyn H. Saiki
113 Sierra Vista Ave.
Apt. B
Mountain View, CA 94043
650-965-8105

Mona Salinas
5527 Shattuck Ave.
#306
Oakland, CA 94609
415-948-9501

Katrina Schneider
PO Box 99353
San Diego, CA 92169
858-688-3042

Bonne Schulman-Rust
373 Belmont Ave.
Redwood City, CA 94061
650-368-5997

Wahida Sharman
1070 42nd St.
Sacramento, CA 95819
916-452-2750

Susan Simon
3851 Holland Dr.
Santa Rosa, CA 95404
415-507-0786

Rebecca Slovin
1664 Larkin
Apt. 14
San Francisco, CA 94109
415-771-1627

Emylena Squires
15 Arlington Lane
Kensington, CA 94707
510-835-2200

Dee Stauffer
10190 N. Foothill Expressway
Cupertino, CA 95014
408-737-2031

Leslie Stein
4716 Park Granada
Unit 199
Calabasas, CA 91302
818-954-5023

April Sugarman
1235 Yale St.
Apt. 3
Santa Monica, CA 90404
310-447-0669

Andrea Sulzbacher
1601 Artefia Blvd.
Apt. 4
Manhattan Beach, CA 90266
310-318-9807

Hwee Giok Tan Grace Wu
1186 Maraschino Dr.
Sunnyvale, CA 94087
408-736-6172

Kendi Taylor
3600 Fillmore St.
Apt. 209
San Francisco, CA 94123
415-463-4567

Kathleen Tompkins
929 Idaho Ave.
Apt. 2
Santa Monica, CA 90403
310-234-8921

Kelly Tourgeman
2438 Lyric Ave.
Los Angeles, CA 90027
323-913-1810

Keegan Tyler
862 S. Catalina St.
Los Angeles, CA 90005
818-842-4384

Haley Alexander Vanoosten
PO Box 24297
Los Angeles, CA 90024
310-473-0904

Kathy Ward
1081 Harrington Way
Carmichael, CA 95608
916-486-3859

Deborah Watkins
5000 Centinella
Los Angeles, CA 90066
310-398-4006

Ashlee Wilcox
1303 Manhattan Beach Blvd.
Manhattan Beach, CA 90266
310-376-4886

Jennifer Wilson
19524 Nordhoff St.
Apt. 8B
Northridge, CA 91324
818-713-1518

Aggie Winston
4550 Tam O'Shanter Dr.
Westlake Village, CA 91362
805-373-1440

Sarah Wise
2384 Dartmouth
Redding, CA 96001
530-247-1450

Brianna Wollenweber
2255 Showers Dr.
#164
Mountain View, CA 94040
650-559-0622

**Colorado**

Kim Barry
8279 E. 28th Pl.
Denver, CO 80238
303-386-3636

Lynne Brown
1125 S. Gilpin St.
Denver, CO 80210
303-733-5664

Christa Dunbar
2224 S. Pinon Court
Denver, CO 80210
303-984-2183

Sarah Elson
1101 Colorado Blvd.
#4
Denver, CO 80206
303-905-4959

Lauren Gillespie
PO Box 134
Trinidad, CO 81082
719-680-2440

Elizabeth Ikard
1300 W. Stuart St.
#16
Fort Collins, CO 80526
970-472-8699

Asia Jenkins
PO Box 11502
Aspen, CO 81612
970-948-5849

Michelle Kenney
1859 Meadow Ridge Rd.
Unit B
Vail, CO 81657
970-480-0405

Dana Lindley
8016 S. Vine Way
Littleton, CO 80122
303-734-0033

Heather Marinaccio
Boulder, CO 80302
303-280-1415

Wendy Moore
PO Box 6690
Snowmass Village, CO 81615
970-379-4194

Suzie Poetsch
PO Box 1441
Fraser, CO 80442
719-481-1368

Wendy Puckett
Steamboat Pilates and Fitness Studio
PO Box 881657
Steamboat Springs, CO 80488
970-871-1313

Pam Reitan
5438 S. Swadley Court
Littleton, CO 80127
303-933-7601

Sarah Smysor
1041 Ogden St.
#201
Denver, CO 80218
303-860-1460

Lisa Tanguma
6640 E. 73rd Pl.
Commerce City, CO 80022
303-289-4588

Natalie Taylor
3840 Fox St.
Englewood, CO 80110
303-668-0467

Margaret Teixeira
0063 Ute Ave.
Carbondale, CO 81623
303-440-5776

Jacqueline Trombly
198 Eastwood Rd.
Aspen, CO 81611
719-440-2861

Tina Tucker
333 Lamprecht Dr.
Carbondale, CO 81623
970-704-0882

Ryan White
23681 Broadmoor Dr.
Parker, CO 80138
720-851-0605

**Connecticut**

Diane Black
21 Prospect Rd.
Westport, CT 06880
203-227-5188

Alison Bricken
98 South Compo Rd.
Westport, CT 06880
203-222-2287

Liz Clingham
351 Pemberwick Rd.
Unit 705
Greenwich, CT 06831
203-531-6826

Charlene Erwin
38 Pumpkin Hill Rd.
Westport, CT 06880
203-226-2686

Justine Fuller
36 Sherman St.
#2F

Hartford, CT 06105
860-232-7469

Diana Hooker
61 N. Mountain Rd.
Brookfield, CT 06804
203-740-1743

Karen Kopf
581 Roosevelt Dr.
Oxford, CT 06478
203-734-1776

Babette Lienhard
23 Riverbank Rd.
Weston, CT 06883
203-227-2291

Margherita Shaw
111 Pilfershire Rd.
Eastford, CT 06242-9472
860-255-5268

Keri Simoson
4 Nappa Lane
Westport, CT 06880
203-226-1389

Sandy Young Bodyworks
Attn: Sandy Young
645 Post Rd. E.
Westport, CT 06880
203-226-3401

## District of Columbia

Barbara Bush
3502 McKinley St. NW
Washington, DC 20015
202-362-0415

S. Kaye Gardner
4339 Massachusetts Ave. NW
Washington, DC 20016
202-237-8211

Susan Perry
1824 47th Pl. NW
Washington, DC 20007
202-338-3339

Arja Pirinen
1801 Clydesdale Place NW #503
Washington, DC 20009
202-234-0304

## Delaware

Nancy Hawkins
PO Box 44
Camden, DE 19934
302-674-5600

## Florida

Alecia-Jane Elizabeth Arts
2865 Wild Lake Blvd.
Pensacola, FL 32526
850-941-2807

Kiomara Atkinson
5433 Lynn Lake Dr.
St. Petersburg, FL 33712
727-897-9146

Lore Ayoub
936½ 17th Ave. NE
St. Petersburg, FL 33704
727-236-3457

Catherine Bedard
4210 W. San Pedro St.
Tampa, FL 33629
813-908-6053

Colleen Blankenship-Borgo
15150 NW 6th Court
Pembroke Pines, FL 33028
786-208-3311

Christine Borchers
19309 Pierpoint Court
Lutz, FL 33558
813-948-4908

Donna Boyer
8759 Crestgate Circle
Orlando, FL 32819
407-876-6333

Lisa Daniel
4324 S. Kirkman Rd.
Orlando, FL 32811
407-294-9333

Melissa Dann
2620 4th St. N.
St. Petersburg, FL 33704
727-525-5103

Elizabeth DeMarse
13028 Tall Pine Circle
Fort Myers, FL 33907
239-240-8088

Denise Dorney
796 Summit Lake Dr.
West Palm Beach, FL 33406
561-809-3935

Veronica Esteban
7500 NW 25th St.
Miami, FL 33122
305-338-4548

Aurora Farber
379 10th St.
Atlantic Beach, FL 32233
904-241-3825

Linda Gelcich
4819 Okara Rd.
Tampa, FL 33617
813-985-7068

Cassandra Giddens
9927 Brassie Bend
Naples, FL 34108
239-514-3375

Jehna Johnson
9521 Raptor Court
Tallahassee, FL 32308
850-877-0247

Amanda Koch
316 Cherry St.
#35
Panama City, FL 32401
850-747-3881

Athena Liolios
713 E. Golf Blvd.
Indian Rock Beach, FL 33785
727-596-0089

Karen Mirlenbrink
330 Promenade Dr.
#207
Dunedin, FL 34698
727-736-9309

Brandy Price
1045 9th Ave. N.
St. Petersburg, FL 33705
727-455-1753

Mireya Prio
10380 Vanderbilt Dr.
Naples, FL 34108
239-597-1075

Maressa Rahn
4732 S. Kirkman Rd.
Orlando, FL 32811
407-293-9200

Traci Roshitsh-Weems
10701 Cleary Blvd.
Apt. 106
Plantation, FL 33324
954-781-2984

Alison Schiltz
5971 Westgate Dr.
Apt. 1222
Orlando, FL 32835
407-313-1939

Vicki Sullivan
2744 Woody Pl.
Jacksonville, FL 32216
904-996-7319

Kristine Belding Toledo
1000 NW Ten Court
Miami, FL 33136
305-324-4397

Catherine Whitehurst
Body Balance of Clearwater
1221 N. Cleveland St.
Clearwater, FL 33755
727-452-3251

Roberta Zemo
15 NE 11th St.
Delray Beach, FL 33444
561-274-8593

## Hawaii

Lisa Castelein
1759 B Lawerence Rd.
Kailua, HI 96734
808-253-0014

Jessica Dung
91-1037 Makaaloa St.
Ewa Beach, HI 96707
808-371-4389

Carmen Ferri
264 Kawailani Circle
Kihei
Maui HI 96753
808-879-3260

Mia Howard
45-934 Kam Hwy.
#C125
Kaneohe, HI 96744
808-521-1316

Theresa Ouano
PO Box 770
Kalaheo, HI 96741
808-332-0616

Pam Sandridge
309 Anolani St.
Honolulu, HI 96821
808-373-5175

## Idaho

Brian Kelly
PO Box 4474
Ketchum, ID 83340
208-720-2736

## Illinois

Eme Cole
Pilates Plus
504 W. Arlington Pl.
Chicago, IL 60614
773-832-1289

Davi Edelbeck
1029 N. Mozart
Chicago, IL 60622
773-342-9927

Janice Fenske
22724 W. Loon Lake Blvd.
Antioch, IL 60002
847-395-3984

Lauren Fonseca
2984 Acorn Lane
Northbrook, IL 60062
847-858-2722

Kim Gore
913 Rollingwood Road
Highland Park, IL 60035
773-883-1444

Geraldine Gremlich-Sherk
2308 Old Hicks Rd.
Palatine, IL 60067
773-665-1070

Kathy Jacques
25 Ronan Rd.
#206
Highwood, IL 60040
847-209-0324

Jean Kind
1205 W. Sherwin
Apt. 502
Chicago, IL 60626
312-409-3300

Katy Lush
617 W. Surf St.
#4
Chicago, IL 60657
312-672-9610

Lisa Sullivan
2104 E. Pennsylvania
Urbana, IL 61802
217-367-9707

Maureen Twohey
1430 W. Maude
Arlington Heights, IL 60004
847-392-4932

## Indiana

Karen Falloon
12517 Timber Creek Dr.
#10
Carmel, IN 46032
317-672-8777

Kathy Levine
13532 Spring Farms Dr.
Carmel, IN 46032
317-571-1211

Kara Reibel
10427 Athalene Lane
McCordsville, IN 46055-9622
317-590-5558

Stacey Valant
Pilates Center Indianapolis, Inc.
176 E. Carmel Dr.
Carmel, IN 46032
317-571-1137

Andrea Wilson
7136 Westminster Dr.
Indianapolis, IN 46256
317-849-2416

## Kansas

Margot Gray
1903 Quail Creek Dr.
Lawrence, KS 66047
785-843-1717

## Kentucky

Pamela Barnhart
1411 S. 4th St.
Louisville, KY 40208

Kimberly Cox
331 Kenilworth Rd.
Apt. 1
Louisville, KY 40206
502-899-1181

Claire Greenlee
1805 Stevens Ave.
Louisville, KY 40205
502-456-5778

Gloria Lawrence-Rangel
309 N. Main St.
Lexington, KY 24450
859-461-3447

Francie Mulloy
2015 Camargo Rd.
Louisville, KY 40207
502-896-2629

## Louisiana

Carol Conway
306 S. French Quarter Dr.
Houma, LA 70364
504-872-6185

Kristie Guidry
100 Credeur Rd.
Scott, LA 70583
337-873-2183

Jennifer Sloan
645 Rosa Ave.
Metairie, LA 70005
504-236-0041

Kathleen Wiener
4443 Richmond Ave.
Shreveport, LA 71106
318-868-7030

## Maryland

Lizette Ayala
6135 Mountaindale Rd.
Thurmont, MD 21788
301-826-0277

Linda Baum
9402 Balfour Dr.
Bethesda, MD 20814
301-530-6926

Susanna Chase-Burlace
1563 Ritchie Lane
Annapolis, MD 21401
410-263-3766

Deborah Lu
1030 Chinaberry Dr.
Frederick, MD 21703
301-540-3719

Maya Rhinewine
2912 Lindell Court
Silver Spring, MD 20902
301-942-5917

Carla Rosenthal
6631 London Lane
Bethesda, MD 20817
301-229-2092

## Massachusetts

Michelle Adams
91 Appleton Ave.
Pittsfield, MA 01201
508-469-9960

Kathleen Currie
5 Wood St.
Middleboro, MA 02346
508-946-1891

Pamela Garcia
42 Carriage Rd.
Hanson, MA 02341
781-826-9539

Reed Kream
102 Cliff Rd.
Milton, MA 02186
617-696-8910

Joan McKenney
102 Pine St.
Quincy, MA 02170
617-872-3152

Gail Rosier
30 Lyman St.
Westborough, MA 01581
508-579-5588

Sandy Salvucci
502 Hosmer St.
Marlboro, MA 01752
508-229-7864

Diana Tubbs
Mount Auburn Club
Attn: Faryl Norris
57 Coolidge Ave.
Watertown, MA 02472
617-926-3052

## Michigan

Melissa Francis
35255 Rhonswood Dr.
Farmington Hills, MI 48335
734-623-8511

Nancy Meier
3551 Windemere Dr.
Ann Arbor, MI 48105
734-388-5855

Judith Veliquette
14537 Spirea Dr.
Elk Rapids, MI 49629
231-264-5254

## Minnesota

Sara Bolier
3700 41st Ave. S.
Minneapolis, MN 55406
612-729-6656

Debra Dodge
19700 Schutte Farm Rd.
Corcoran, MN 55340
763-416-1388

Sharon Picasso-Merrick
612 8th Ave. N.
South St. Paul, MN 55075
612-600-4903

## Mississippi

Sherry Hager
230 Garden St.
Ridgeland, MS 39157
601-605-0841

## Montana

Kirsten Quande-Cherubini
2620 Park St.
Missoula, MT 59803
406-251-2963

Natalie Swanson
PO Box 8119
Bozeman, MT 59773
406-240-9238

## New Hampshire

Sharon Barry
Rte. 101A
Amherst, NH 03031
603-578-0282

## New Jersey

Tammy Campbell
2 Hanover Court
Bordentown, NJ 08505
609-291-9495

Marlo DeNapoli
500 Second St.
Dunellen, NJ 08812
732-968-9025

Connie Fazekas
32 Steeple Chase Court
Asbury, NJ 08802
908-537-1147

Tegan Fischer
112 14th St.
#2
Hoboken, NJ 07030
201-946-5236

Heather Garman
1512 Garden Dr.
Apt. 12
Ocean, NJ 07712
732-493-4533

Cheryl Giballa
9721 Second Ave.
Stone Harbor, NJ 08247
732-487-0321

Rosanne Knabe
9 Marigold Lane
Califon, NJ 07830
908-832-3010

Michelle Margolin
337 Franklin St.
Haworth, NJ 07641
201-567-8753

Deborah Price
JCC of Central Jersey
1391 Martine Ave.
Scotch Plains, NJ 07076
908-322-2960

Lisa Waldman
57-19 Bridgewaters Dr.
Oceanport, NJ 07757
732-389-2728

## New Mexico

Kelly Higgins
1548 16th Ave.
Rio Rancho, NM 87124
505-891-9048

Hallie Love
1409 Santa Rosa
Santa Fe, NM 87505
505-986-0994

Rachael Penn
312 A Burch St.
Taos, NM 87571
505-751-1590

## New York

Gail Accardi
15 Stuyvesant Oval
Apt. 12 G
New York, NY 10009
212-995-8089

Erika Bloom
9 Stanton St.
#5A
New York, NY 10002
646-602-9649

Angelique Christensen
19 Nassau St.
Plainview, NY 11803
516-827-9389

Michael Feigin
512 Bedford Rd.
Armonk, NY 10504
914-273-8922

Carolyn Giacalone
752 West End Ave.
Apt. 15-F
New York, NY 10025
212-875-4018

Lawson Harris
512 Bedford Rd.
Armonk, NY 10504
914-273-8922 or 917-751-0393

Elizabeth Hart
100 Stanton St.
#3B
New York, NY 10002
212-539-0132

Christina Huber
1 Van Houten St.
Upper Nyack, NY 10960
845-358-7432

Olga Jabbour
5 Nassau Blvd.
Garden City, NY 11530
516-739-2184

Shauna Jenkisson
231 14th St.
Brooklyn, NY 11215
917-582-0677

Tonia Johnson
PO Box 608
Mount Vernon, NY 10552
914-841-6344

Angela Jones
68-12 Yellowstone Blvd.
Forest Hills, NY 11375
917-686-7178

Pat Kostikerich
55 Montauk Ave.
Central Islip, NY 11722
631-665-4645

Camille Leon
32 Continental Rd.
Warwick, NY 10990
845-988-0258

Lavinia Long
53 W. 106th St.
Apt. 2A
New York, NY 10025
212-866-8552

Tracie Matthews
414 Degraw St.
Brooklyn, NY 11231
718-330-9641

Denise Miller
25 Royal Oaks Ave.
Middletown, NY 10940
845-386-8086

Molly Phelps
144 W. 109th St.
#2E
New York, NY 10025

Lauren Piskin
1725 York Ave.
#11F
New York, NY 10125
212-876-8424

Janessa Rick
101 W. 23rd St.
#2401
New York, NY 10011
917-353-2412

Lisa Smilkstein
10 S. Beechwood Rd.
Bedford Hills, NY 10507
914-666-3763

Nanako Ueda
144 Fourth Ave.
#3
Brooklyn, NY 11217
718-399-9443

**North Carolina**

Leigh Brown
PO Box 52
Saxapahaw, NC 27340
336-376-0836

Rachel Brown
200 Oak Pine Dr.
Apex, NC 27502
919-363-8676

Stacie Dombrowski
206 Lewey Brook Dr.
Cary, NC 27519
919-363-0556

Patricia (Patty) Geiger
102 N. Coslett Ct.
Cary, NC 27513
919-460-5332

Missy Grant
10813 Cokesbury Lane
Raleigh, NC 27615
919-466-0982

Margarita Hadisurya
c/o Blane Lewis CID/RTI
PO Box 12194
Research Triangle Park, NC
    27709-2194
919-769-5173

Susan Heath
8504 Clivedon Dr.
Raleigh, NC 27615
919-870-6655

Alice Jackson
2233 Noble Rd.
Raleigh, NC 27608
919-832-7642

Nina Jonson
10416 Veasey Mill Rd.
Raleigh, NC 27615
919-846-3785

Mark Kosiewski
1025 Holly Creek Lane
Chapel Hill, NC 27516
919-969-7740

Julie Mills
Northstone Country Club
15801 Northstone Dr.
Huntersville, NC 28078
704-671-7672

Sarah Tauber
7100 Brandemere Lane
Apt. E
Winston-Salem, NC 27106
336-767-8518

## Ohio

Michelle Bump
5620 Whitney Pl.
Cincinnati, OH 45227
513-271-2911

Antonia Galdos
58 Hereford St.
Cincinnati, OH 45216
513-761-6325

Vanessa Jay
556 Wiltshire St.
Apt. A
Dayton, OH 45419

Douglas Lenser
1200 Blind Brook Dr.
Columbus, OH 43235
614-846-2339

Fiona Taylor
8530 Cornett's Cove
Maineville, OH 45039
513-706-0309

Mary Willis
5251 Longshadow Dr.
Westerville, OH 43081-7827
614-855-2196

## Oklahoma

Ros Elder
5205 S. Yorktown Ave.
Tulsa. OK 74105
918-747-0735

## Oregon

Tracy Broyles
1307 SE 17th St.
Portland, OR 97214
503-233-6764

Wendy Bucko
2006 SE 32nd Pl.
Portland, OR 97214
503-239-4270

Daniel Epstein
1630 SE 41st Ave.
Portland, OR 97202
503-658-3899

Gina Frabotta
2124 NE Davis St.
Portland, OR 97232
503-239-6218

Joelle Miller
9542 SW Jonathan Court
Portland, OR 97219
503-768-9799

Christina Sproule
PO Box 455
Hood River, OR 97031
541-386-2105

Gina Stierlin
2008 Virginia Lane
West Linn, OR 97068
503-780-0771

Kathryn Todd
3126 SE 22nd St.
Portland, OR 97202
503-239-6041

## Pennsylvania

Megan Armitage
balanCenter Pilates
915 Montgomery Ave.
Suite 305
Narberth, PA 19072
215-271-7855

Christy Bradberry
PO Box 374
Macungie, PA 18062
610-393-2500

Eileen Erlich
1553 Grovania Ave.
Abington, PA 19001
215-657-6576

Mary Ewart
Spring and Spiral
5824 Forbes Ave.
Pittsburgh, PA 15217
412-472-2401

Adina Filipoi
12 Village Lane
Bethany, PA 18431
570-971-7443

Margie Foley
536 Ashbourne Rd.
Cheltenham, PA 19012
267-978-1478

Elizabeth Gelesky
1221 Marlborough St.
Philadelphia, PA 19125
215-423-2326

Linda Houck
Pilates by Linda
2727 Philmont Ave.
Suite 132
Huntingdon Valley, PA 19006
215-947-5058 or 215-947-5510

Joanna McLaughlin
485 A. Kirk Lane
Media, PA 19063
610-892-4919

Sarah Orlowitz
507 Haverford Ave.
Narberth, PA 19072
215-667-7854

Jeff Prall
321 N. Front St.
Apt. 2G
Philadelphia, PA 19106
215-629-1108

Andrea Sapiente
1561 Watson St.
Williamsport, PA 17701
570-745-3139

Ruth Way
3408 Midvale Ave.
Philadelphia, PA 19129
215-882-3690

Geri Weatherholtz
211 Wellington Ave.
West Lawn, PA 19609
610-777-7914

### Rhode Island

Deanna Potts
43 King St.
East Greenwich, RI 02818
401-885-6819

Tim Robertson
106 Canton St.
1st Floor
Providence, RI 02908
401-274-1465

Bill Wilson
171 Modena Ave.
Providence, RI 02908
401-454-7612

Lindsey Yates
45 Princess Pine Dr.
East Greenwich, RI 02818
401-885-0423

### Texas

Stephanie Atkinson
2002 Forest Park Blvd.
#8
Fort Worth, TX 76110
817-481-9345

Bernice Baca-Vigil
6074 Tanglewood Trail
Spring Branch, TX 78070-5245
830-228-5347

Cathi Brown
1319 West Gray
Houston, TX 77019
713-523-6842

Frances Caron
PO Box 324
Washington, TX 77880
936-878-2480

Roxanne D'Ascenzo-Hawkins
45 Scotsmoor Court
Sugarland, TX 77479
281-565-6944

Maureen Dunn
4141 Rosemead Pkwy
#5301
Dallas, TX 75287
214-741-9274

Leslie Ervin
4606 Horseshoe Bend
Austin, TX 78731
512-459-7926

Stephanie Hahn
7501 Bella Vista Trail
Austin, TX 78737
512-301-8734

Kristie Kiser
6528 Haskell
Houston, TX 77007
713-227-1583

Kathy McCann
9417 OSR
Midway, TX 75852
512-358-7186

Cindy Nelson
8004 Danforth Cove
Austin, TX 78746
512-328-5839

Diane Pulos
298 Sugarberry Circle
Houston, TX 77024
713-781-0462

Brooke Reece
4203 Bradwood Rd.
Austin, TX 78722
512-453-0313

Amy Stanley
3303 W. Creek Club Dr.
Missouri City, TX 77459
281-261-5934

Sabrina Swayder
1710 Maryland
#1
Houston, TX 77006
713-942-9941

Jacqueline Todd
3808 El Campo
Ft. Worth, TX 76107
817-791-5047

Jana Watts
Fitness Quest Studio
108 North Ave. E.
Suite 203
Bryan, TX 77801
979-693-2406

**Virginia**

Kathleen Boisvert
11710 Rockaway Lane
Fairfax, VA 22030
703-502-9680

Bonnie Bowers
3797 Center Way
Fairfax, VA 22033
703-352-5436

Leila Conklin
PO Box 41776
Arlington, VA 22204
703-683-9815

Jennifer Corney
5008 Grimm Dr.
Alexandria, VA 22304
703-823-1122

Debra Edgell
9514 Draycott Court
Burke, VA 22015
703-249-9478

Kathleen Faris
2110 N. Pierce St.
#7
Arlington, VA 22209-1118
703-243-2262

Jackie Martin
604 River Rd.
Newport News, VA 23601
757-599-0928

Kara Martucci
43175 Center St.
Chantilly, VA 20152
703-591-5951

Pam McGeorge
3112 Rendale Ave.
Richmond, VA 23221
804-358-5343

Madeline Parrish
325 Ryefield Rd.
Richmond, VA 23233
804-784-5659

Elizabeth Penn
3704 L Steeplechase Way
Williamsburg, VA 23188
757-540-1458

Gerry Stowers
219 W. Beverley St.
Suite 206
Staunton, VA 24401
540-255-2182

Nadine Tyreman
7901 Belmont Court
Marshall, VA 20115
540-364-4689

## Washington

Santee Brewster
1005 Pine Ave. NE
Olympia, WA 98506
360-352-2119

Michelle Hoyos
126 214th St. SE
Bothell, WA 98021
360-402-0465

Rose (Elaine) McFarlane
2281 Uscandia Lane
Point Roberts, WA 98281
360-945-2342

Brook Visser
584 King Fisher Lane
Friday Harbor, WA 98250
360-601-8558

## Wisconsin

Sheri Baemmert
4913 River Glen Court
Eau Claire, WI 54703
715-559-8861

Susan Hogg
1535 Red Oak Court
Middleton, WI 53562
608-831-1051

Andrea West Dow
3451 N. Frederick Ave.
Milwaukee, WI 53211
262-853-4882

## Bermuda

Kristina Ingham
PO Box HM 2140
Hamilton, HMJX
441-292-2192

## Canada

## Alberta

Tara Bennett
10736 69th Ave.
Edmonton, Alberta T6H 2E1

## Ontario

Melissa Cedrone
3082 Line 6
RR1
Bradford, ON L3Z 2A4
905-775-5895

Jennifer Coyne
40 Park Rd.
Apt. 506
Toronto, ON M4W 2N4
416-972-9994

Lori Dunn
97 Douglas Ave.
Toronto, ON M5M 1G4
416-485-5607

Anjelee French
2 Southhampton St.
Guelph, ON N1H 5N4
519-763-2464

Victoria Gardiner
195 Galaxy Blvd.
Etobicoke, ON M9W 6R7
416-674-7809

Pamela Knight
5915 Tampico Way
Mississauga, ON L5M 6V3
905-821-3792

Susan Lee
University of Toronto
55 Harbord St.
Toronto, ON M5S 2W6
416-979-1654

Stacey Martin
37 Nestow Dr.
Ottawa, ON K2G 4M2
705-609-6840

Regina Radisic
550 Jarvis St.
Apt. 320
Toronto, ON M4Y 2H9
416-927-8845

Dawn Wells
45 Maydolph Rd.
Toronto, ON M9B 1W2
416-626-6333

## Colombia

Maria Clara Ramirez Roa
Calle 86
#764
Apt. 501
Bogota
571-211-2901

## England

Sandrine Lindsay
1a Park Hill Rd.
Orana, Kent TN14 5QH
11-85229879422

## Indonesia

Fransisca Hadisurya Jalan Saraswati
    Ujung
No. 1
Cipete Utara Jakarta 12150
62217254433

## Japan

Momoko Takanashi
1-29-13 Komone Itabashi-ku
Tokyo
173-212-3751362

# Glossary

**alignment**   State of physical being that establishes and maintains the natural lineup of the skeletal structure.

**ankle foundation**   Good alignment of the ankle joint over the foot.

**bowing**   Movement of the upper spine only in a lengthened forward flexion indicated by a softening of the breastbone.

**bridging**   Lifting of the pelvis, with neutral spine, off the floor using legs from a supine position (lying on your back) with your feet on the floor and knees bent.

**cat**   Spinal extension and flexion exercise on all fours, or two hands and two knees.

**cervical spine**   The seven vertebrae between your shoulders and occiput.

**conscious breathing**   Inhalation facilitates torso extension and rotation; exhalation facilitates torso flexion. Proper breathing efficiently directs muscular activation and engagement; conscious breathing promotes focus.

**differentiation**   Movement separation within joints and specific skeletal structures (examples: rib cage and pelvis, head and cervical vertebrae, pelvis and hip joints, etc.).

**extension**   Elongation and opening of the front of the torso while the facet joints of the spine are closing for stability. Extension increases the angle of the joint. This happens in the sagittal plane or front to back.

**femur**   Leg bone between the pelvis and the knee.

**first position**   Hip open, legs and heels touching, and feet turned out in a small V.

**flexion**   Shortening, folding, or bending movement at the joint where bones move closer together.

**gluteus maximus**   Outside layer and largest butt muscle. It attaches to the outer upper leg and the middle of the lowest part of the back. Pulls the thigh bones backward.

**hamstrings**   Three muscles in the back of the legs that run from the sitting bones down to the back of the knees. Assist the glutes in pulling the thigh bones backward.

**hip extension**   Lengthening in front of the hip by using the muscles in the back of the leg.

**hip rotators**  Move the femur in the hip socket inward and outward.

**humerus**  Bone that extends from the shoulder to the elbow.

**iliopsoas**  Called psoas, it is the muscle that runs from the lumbar vertebrae into the front surface of the pelvis (ilium), then down to the inner upper legs (lesser trochanter) at the groin. Bends the hip joints, bringing the legs toward the pelvis.

**ischial tuberosity**  One of the three bones that make up the pelvis. Also known as the sitting bones.

**lateral flexion**  Side bending of the spine, left or right.

**lateral shift**  Shifting the pelvis sideways using your leg.

**lumbar spine**  Vertebrae between the lowest rib and the pelvis.

**mobilization**  Movement in a joint or specific segment of the body; accompanied by stabilizing one end of a joint so that mobilization occurs at the other end.

**neutral spine**  Position that allows the spine to find natural placement. Precluding any flexion or extension movement, the shape of the spine from head to tail effortlessly maintains spinal curves but is individually different from one person to the next. Relates to the plumb line between the top of the spine in the head through the tailbone through the center of the head.

**obliques (internal and external)**  Side and waistline muscles that run from the side of the ribs diagonally to the top of the pelvic bones (ilium); internal fibers wrap posteriorly; external fibers wrap anteriorly. Their functions include inside bending and rotation.

**occiput**  Rear section of the head or skull.

**pectoral muscles (pecs)**  Muscles in front of the chest that assist in lifting the arms.

**pelvic floor/abdominal engagement**  Accessing and engaging muscles between the pubis and tail in an upward internal motion coupled with narrowing inward of the deep abdominal (transversus abdominis) muscles to stabilize the pelvis and lower back.

**pelvis**  Hip bones.

**pike**  A position in which the hands and feet are on the floor and the base of the spine is lifted so that the torso and the hands form a triangle.

**plié**  A position involving bending of the knees.

**prolapse**  A condition in which the uterus, the bladder, the bowel, or all three drop downward in the pelvis below their normal positions.

**proprioception**   The unconscious perception of movement and special orientation arising from stimuli within the body itself.

**pubis**   Pubic bone.

**quadriceps**   Large muscles in front of the thigh bones.

**rectus abdominis**   Major belly muscle ("six-pack abs") running from the front of the rib cage down to the pubic bone. Bends the torso forward.

**releve**   A position in which the weight moves to the toes so the heels lift and the body rises up.

**retraction**   Moving the shoulder girdle and blades together toward the vertebral column.

**rib cage connection**   Relaxes and softens the front of the ribs.

**rotation**   Motion around a central axis that is activated in the transverse plane (horizontal). Rotation is also circumduction, a circular movement of a bone in a joint (circumduction involves flexors, extensors, adductors, and abductors) that is activated in all planes.

**sacrum**   Triangular bone in the back of the pelvis that features fused vertebrae of the lower spine before the tailbone.

**scapulae**   Also known as the shoulder blades, these are the bones that make up the back of the shoulders.

**serratus anterior**   Large banana bunch muscle (like fingers) attaches to the inner edge (vertebral border) of the shoulder blades (near the spine) and fans out around the upper ribs. Assists in upward rotation of the outer tip of the shoulder blades.

**spinal sequencing**   Articulation of the vertebral column affected by engaging abdominal muscles in flexion and/or posterior muscles in extension.

**stabilization**   Muscles that stabilize are found in the trunk/core of the body. Awareness and recruitment of these muscles will allow increased range of motion in extremity joints as well as prevention of trauma or injury around the spine and vertebrae.

**sternum**   Breastbone; long, flat bone connected to the first seven ribs.

**swan**   A prone position in which the head and shoulders are extended and the heart is lifted up.

**thorax**   Section of the body that contains the heart and lungs; the chest.

**torso rotation**   Motion around a central axis that includes the lumbar, thoracic, and cervical spine. It is initiated by the deep spinal muscles and further activated by the extrinsic trunk muscles.

**transversus abdominis**   A horizontal muscle that acts as a corset between the ribs and the hips. It keeps your internal organs in place.

**trapezius**   Two triangular muscles that run from the base of the occipus to the middle of the back.

**trunk**   Torso, area between the shoulders and hip joints.

**tuck**   Squeezing of buttocks to push the hips forward, which flexes the spine.

**turn-out**   Outward rotation of the leg in the hip socket.

**V arms**   Shape of the arms held overhead and the importance of wide shoulder blades to support them.

# Index

abdominals
    and breathing, 9, 24–25, 50, 52
    in the Foundations, 22
    in the Fundamentals, 9, 11–12,
        14, 19–21
    in the mat exercises, 30–32,
        34–35, 38–39, 40–41
    in the Standing Exercises, 52, 79
alcohol, and osteoporosis, 154, 156,
    159
alignment
    analyzing, 45
    of the domes, 25
    of the head, 38, 103
    of the hips, 38–39, 71
    importance of, 44, 59
    of the knees and ankles, 59, 67,
        71, 83, 103
    of the legs, 59, 83, 99, 103
    of the pelvis, 63, 107, 131
    of the rib cage, 38, 71
    of the shoulders, 67, 75, 91
    in Single–Leg Foundation, 50,
        115
    of the spine, 39, 91
    in Spine Twist, 87
    in the Teaser, 115
ankles, alignment of, 67, 83, 103
Arm Circles, 19
Arm Foundation, 50
Arm Fundamentals, 17–19, 50

arms
    activating, 59, 83
    in dynamic sitting, 144
    lengthening, 101
    relation to back, 67, 83
    relation to shoulders, 17–18,
        54–55, 75, 119, 123
    rotation of, 55
    and spinal rotation, 91
    weight–bearing, 99, 127, 139
awareness
    increasing, 8, 22, 67, 111
    in the Pilates Method, 4
    of position, 44–45
    in Standing Exercises, 50–51, 139
    watching others, 45–46

back. *See also* spine
    arms' relation to, 83
    extension of, 41
    in Front Fundamentals, 19–21
balance
    and alignment, 71
    brain compensating for closed
        eyes in, 46, 71
    influences on, 55, 103
    in standing exercises, 44, 55, 59,
        71, 103, 111, 119
Balanchine, George, 152
Bartenieff, Irmagard, 7
blood disorders, and bone loss, 155

bone marrow disorders, and bone loss, 155

bones
increasing density of, 153–154, 156
loss of density in, 154–155
source of changes in, 156–158

Bow, the, 25, 50
in the Neck Pull, 105–107
in the Single–Leg Stretch, 30, 69, 71

brain
compensating for closed eyes, 46, 71
effects of head position on, 142
Fundamentals and Foundations to train, 46–47, 144

breathing
abdominals and, 34, 52
diaphragm in, 24–25, 36–37
importance of, 55, 75
lifting domes through, 24–25
percussive, 55
in the standing exercises, 46–47, 50, 55, 123
in Torso Fundamentals, 9

Bridging, 15–16

calcium, and bone loss, 153–154, 156–157

cancers, and bone loss, 155–156

Cat, the, 20–21, 41

choreography, 67
of the standing exercises, 49, 91

Contrology, 4

Corkscrew, the, 88–91

Cushing's syndrome, and bone loss, 155

daily movements
knee alignment in, 83
rib rotation in, 37
standing exercises as, 51
as whole–body vs. partial, 27

Dance Notation Bureau, 7

diaphragm, 44
in breathing, 36–37
as dome, 24–25

diet
and osteoporosis, 158–159
and weight loss, 46

Domes, the
aligning, 25–27
in feet, 22
lifting, 24–25, 26, 50, 59, 87
while sitting, 141, 143

Double–Leg Kick, 40–42

Double–Leg Stretch, 72–75

dynamic sitting, 143–144

eating
awareness of, 46
disorders of, 155

energizing, 45–46, 111

estrogen, and osteoporosis, 154, 156–158

eyes, and balance, 46, 55, 71

feet
alignment of, 71, 115
awareness of, 54–55, 107
dome of, 25

in the Standing Foundation, 22
Feldenkrais, 7–8
Flight, 19–20
form, of Standing Pilates, 49–50
Foundations, the, 22–27
    goals of, 22, 46
    in standing exercises, 50
Front Fundamentals, 19–21
Fundamentals, the
    arm, 17–19
    development of, 8
    front, 19–21
    goals of, 8, 46
    head, 16–17
    leg, 11–16
    Standing. *See* Foundations, the
    in standing exercises, 50
    torso, 8–11

gender, and bone density, 153, 156
Gentry, Eve, 2, 7–8
Graham, Martha, 152
Green, Penelope, 2

hamstrings
    in Leg Fundamentals, 13
    modifications for tight, 37, 39,
        63, 95, 99
    in the Teaser, 115
head, in ideal postures, 142
Head Float, 16–17, 144
Head Fundamental, 16–17
Hip Extension, 20
hips
    alignment of, 23–24, 38–39, 59,
        71

fractures of, 153, 156
lengthening, 40, 99
rotation of, 91
in sitting, 142–144
Hundred, the, 52–55
hyperparathyroidism, and bone loss,
    155–156
hyperthyroidism, and bone loss, 155
hypogonadism, and bone loss, 154,
    156

iliopsoas, in Leg Fundamentals, 11
incontinence, 44
injuries, 7
Institute for the Pilates Method, 2–3,
    151

joints, and alignment, 44

Kicks, 128–131
Klinefelter's syndrome, and bone
    loss, 155
Knee Fold, 11–12, 14, 30, 50
    in dynamic sitting, 144
    in Single–Leg Stretch, 69–71
Knee Stir, 12
Knee Sway, 14–15
knees, 41
    alignment of, 59, 67, 71, 83, 103

Laban, Rudolph, 7
language, to trigger responses, 50
Larsson, Michele, 2
lateral shifts, 83
Leg Circles, 56–59
Leg Fundamentals, 11–16

Leg Kick–Back, 100–103
Leg Pull–Back, 120–123
Leg Slide, 13–14, 50
legs
    alignment of, 59, 83, 99, 103
    crossed, 142
    Fundamentals for, 11–16
    in ideal sitting posture, 142
    kicking, 131
    lengthening, 36, 78–79
    relation between, 83
    relation to abdominals, 39
    relation to pelvis, 38, 63, 79
    relation to spine, 91, 95, 115,
        131
    weight–bearing, 99, 127, 139

malignancies, and bone loss, 154
mat exercises, Classical Pilates,
        29–42
    vs. Standing Pilates, 44
medications, and osteoporosis risk,
        155
menopause, and osteoporosis, 153,
        157–159
mirrors, for awareness of position,
        44–45
mouth, as dome, 25, 71
movement
    need for frequent, 45, 143–144
    in Pilates Method, 4
    training, 27
movement memory. See muscle
        memory
multifidus, 44
muscle memory, 49, 51, 144

muscles
    deep, 24, 152
    effects of excessive flexion on,
        141–142
    and importance of alignment,
        44
    isolating movement of, 11
    of pelvic floor, 24, 44
    use of deeper, 11, 22, 27

neck
    effects of excessive sitting on,
        142
    flexion of, 50
    in Head Fundamental, 16–17
Neck Pull, 104–107
Neutral Spine, 8–9, 37–38
    in Classic Pilates mat exercises,
        30
    in the Fundamentals, 9, 16
    as ideal posture, 141–142

obliques
    in Leg Fundamentals, 11, 15
    in sitting postures, 142
    in Torso Fundamentals, 11
oophorectomy, and bone loss, 154
Open–Leg Rocker, 80–83
organs, pelvic floor supporting,
        43–44
osteopenia, 154, 158
osteoporosis, 43
    benefits of Pilates to, 153–159
    modifications for, 63
    risk factors for, 155, 158–159
    Web sites on, 159–160

pelvic bowl, in Torso Fundamentals, 9–10
pelvic dome, 24
    engaging, 36, 40
    lifting, 30–31, 34, 79, 99
pelvic floor, 24
    in dynamic sitting, 143
    in the Foundations, 22
    functions of, 43–44
    lifting, 36–38, 79
    sources of damage to, 43–44
Pelvic Foundation, 22, 50
pelvis. See also pelvic bowl; pelvic dome; pelvic floor
    alignment of, 63, 107, 131
    in Leg Fundamentals, 11–15
    legs' relation to, 59, 63, 79
    lengthening, 41
    neutral, 11, 15, 31
    preventing prolapse of, 43–44
    in sitting postures, 142–144
    stability of, 38–39
    in Standing Foundation, 22–23
physical activity, and osteoporosis, 150, 156, 158–159
PhysicalMind Institute, 151
pike position, 99
Pilates, Clara, 2, 151
Pilates, Joseph, 1, 4, 7, 145
    background of, 151
    on method, 3, 152
Pilates instructors, 2, 145
Pilates Method
    benefits of, 3, 152
    Classical Mat exercises of, 29–42

evolution of, 2 (See also Standing Pilates)
    goals of, 3–4, 43
    progressions in, 29, 46–47, 49
    renown of, 145
    Standing vs. Classical Mat, 44
    tenets of, 4, 29, 44
Pilates studios, expansion of, 1–2, 151–152
plank position, 99
posture
    analyzing, 45
    correcting, 43, 141–142
    effects of slumped, 37, 141–142
    excessive flexion in, 141–142
    ideal, 8, 141–142
prayer hands position, 52, 54, 75
pregnancy, and osteoporosis, 156–157
prolapse, prevention of, 43–44
proprioception, 111, 139
    with closed eyes, 46, 71
puberty, and osteoporosis, 154, 156
pubis/pubic bones, 24, 63, 107. See also pelvis
Push–Up, 132–135

race, and osteoporosis, 158–159
Rib Cage Arms, 17–18
ribs/rib cage, 123
    alignment of, 38, 71
    and diaphragm dome, 25, 27, 36
    lifting, 36–37, 67, 107
    rotation of the, 36–37, 84
    shoulders' relation to, 18, 91
    spreading, 30, 107
Roll–Down to Swan, 96–99

Rolling Like a Ball
 lying, 34–35
 standing, 64–67
Roll–Up, the (standing), 60–63
Roll–Up/Roll–Down, 31–33
rotation, 127
 alignment during, 87
 arm, 55
 isolating, 87, 91
 of the pelvis, 10–11
 of the rib cage, 36–37, 84
 of the spine, 27, 36–37, 84–87,
  91, 95
 upper body, 87–90

sacrum, 30, 32
Saw, the, 92–95
sex hormones, and osteoporosis,
 155
sexuality, pelvic floor in, 44
shoulders
 alignment of, 67, 75, 91
 in Arm Fundamentals, 17–19
 arms' relation to, 17–18, 32, 75,
  119, 123
 back's relation to, 54, 75
 effects of excessive sitting on,
  142
 spreading, 32, 54–55
Side Kick, 38–39, 108–111
Single–Leg Foundation, 50, 115,
 131
Single–Leg Stance, the, 23–24
Single–Leg Stretch
 lying, 30–31
 standing, 68–71

Single–Leg–Standing Foundation,
 115
sitting
 correcting posture in, 141–142
 dynamic, 143–144
smart bodies, 4–5, 27, 45
smoking, and osteoporosis, 154
Spinal Arms, 26–27
spinal cord injury, and bone loss, 155
spine. *See also* Neutral Spine
 and abdominals, 30–31, 38
 alignment of, 39, 91
 arms' relation to, 27
 bone loss in, 153
 curves of, 9, 21, 33, 67
 in dynamic sitting, 143–144
 extension of, 40, 103
 flexion and extension of, 20, 41
 flexion of, 25, 32–35, 50, 60–63,
  75
 fractures of, 153
 in Front Fundamentals, 20–21
 in Head Fundamental, 16–17
 head's relation to, 25–26
 isolation of top and bottom, 8,
  87, 91
 legs' relation to, 95, 115, 131
 lengthening, 17, 25–27, 31–32,
  59, 77–78, 95, 115, 131
 rotation of, 27, 36–37, 88–91, 95
 stability of, 31, 39, 44, 115
Spine Stretch (standing), 76–79
Spine Twist, 36–37, 84–87
Standing Foundation, 22–23, 50
Standing Pilates. *See also* specific
  exercise names

awareness in, 50–51
breathing in, 46–47
development of, 43
effects of, 154
levels of, 46, 49
Star, the, 136–139
Swan, Roll–Down to, 96–99
swan position, 97–98
Swimming, 116–119

Teaser, the, 112–115
testosterone, and osteoporosis, 154,
    156, 159
The Method Pilates. *See* Pilates
    Method
torso
    in Front Fundamentals, 20
    lengthening, 40, 50–51, 75, 92
    lift of, 67

neutral, 95
rotation of, 87, 91–92
stability of, 39, 119
Torso Fundamentals, 8–11
transversus muscle, 22, 24, 44
Turner's syndrome, and bone loss,
    155
Twist, the, 124–127

upright position, postural changes
    in, 43

weight loss
    and osteoporosis, 158–159
    through reduced quantities, 46
weight–bearing exercise, 99, 127,
    139
    and osteoporosis, 154
wrists, fractures of, 153